STOP Back Pain!
Kiss Your Back, Neck and Sciatic Nerve Pain Goodbye!

You Don't Have to Live with Chronic Back Pain—There Are Many Options for You!

By Kathi Casey, ERYT, CPI

Cover Design by: Killer Covers

Edited by Ned Moore
MoorePublicityNow.com

This book is informational and not intended nor should it be regarded as medical advice. Please consult your physician before beginning any exercise regimen. The author, designer, publisher and distributor expressly disclaim responsibility for any adverse effects arising from the use or application of the information contained in this book.

Printed in the United States of America

Library of Congress Cataloging-in-Publication Data is available upon request

ISBN 978-1937294045

Praise for Kathi Casey and "STOP Back Pain"

"Your body is naturally designed to heal, regenerate, and be whole. Regardless of how long you've suffered or how many ways you've attempted to "make the pain go away," this book is your stepping stone to changing your life! If you are a person who is currently experiencing back pain or are looking for a way to maintain optimal health, then you've grabbed the right book. Kathi Casey has synthesized and integrated a practical and fun approach for understanding and transforming back pain. I highly recommend this book!"

With Infinite Love and Gratitude,

Dr. Darren R. Weissman
Developer of The LifeLine Technique®
www.drdarrenweissman.com
"Every symptom is a gift in strange wrapping paper."

"I have been to physiotherapy and I have been given all sorts of exercises to try but nothing has ever worked and I just gave up. When I received your email, I thought "why bother, it's just going to be like all the rest" but then something (maybe my guardian angel?!!?!) made me click on the link. You don't know how glad I was when I followed your instructions. The exercise that made the biggest impact was the one lying on your back with your legs on the couch. For the few minutes that I lay like that, there was hardly any pain and as I sit here now typing this message, I feel lighter and a lot more hopeful."

Thea Barendse – South Africa

"I can't tell you how good it feels not to have any leg pain after a year and a half! There aren't words to describe how grateful I am for Kathi's help."

Diann Garner – Maryland

"I'm a dental assistant and after many years of bending over people's mouths, I developed severe neck and shoulder pain. Thanks to the exercises that Kathi Casey showed me, my pain is gone and I can enjoy the things I love to do most – playing with my grandchildren, kayaking and biking! Thanks Kathi!"

Susan Schoenrock – Massachusetts

"Kathi Casey's exercises have really helped me to get rid of my sciatic nerve pain. I have no more pain in my back, legs and buttocks. Only 15 minutes a day and I feel like a new person!"

Jackie Rice - Maryland

"I love to play golf, but there times that I couldn't play because of back pain and I hated that! But since Kathi Casey showed me her exercises to relax and strengthen my back muscles, I hardly ever have that nagging back pain anymore!"

Michael Sinopoli – Massachusetts

Contents

Acknowledgments

This book is dedicated to all of my teachers and mentors. You have inspired and encouraged me and helped me to fill my toolbox with the many natural tools that I now use to help people feel better and live healthier lives. There is no greater gift than caring, loving teachers, and I am grateful to have met each and every one of you.

I am eternally grateful to my children and siblings, who have encouraged and supported me through good times and bad. To "Guru Tim," for always knowing the right thing to say at just the right time; to Mary, for your unique way of pulling the blocks out of me and getting me back on track; to Joe, for inspiring us all through living your dream since childhood; to Pat, whose courage and determination in the face of cancer is most likely another book ☺ Mick and Loretta, you are joy and beauty beyond words.

My dear friend Ned Moore, you have provided a shoulder to cry on, groceries when I was struggling, brilliant marketing ideas, champagne to celebrate each milestone along the way and more patience than I thought possible for any one human being—thank you for being you!

Introduction

Me and My Back Pain

"Learning is a treasure that will follow its owner everywhere."

—Chinese proverb

It was a dark and stormy night... No, that's not how this started, but I've always wanted to start a book that way. Hope I've made you smile because that will start us off on the right foot. Laughter truly is the best medicine!

My story of back pain began one day about ten years ago when I was in my late forties. I walked into the foyer of my childhood home and looked at my reflection in our enormous wall mirror—it's ten feet wide by eight feet high. I mean, I *really* looked at the reflection staring back at me—such a huge mirror reflects back your entire reflection—and I did not like what I saw. The person in the mirror was out-of-shape, overweight, stressed-out and had just "thrown her back out" yet again. What had happened to me? Where did that adventurous, joyful, "outside the box" thinker, who believed anything was possible, go? And who was this crippled old lady in the mirror? Hmmmm...

This moment started a process of looking within that I suppose most of us undergo when we reach a certain age. Intellectually, I knew that the choices I'd made that had brought me to this point were due to patterns and habits that could be changed, but change seemed a daunting task. I could create new habits and make better choices beginning right now, but where would I start?

My first new choice was to sign up for a yoga class offered through the wellness center at my local hospital. That decision changed my life forever. My teacher and mentor, Mary Ellen Steveling, so inspired me that a few months later, I made another big change. I sold the bed-and-breakfast I had owned and operated singlehandedly for two years. At the same time, I resigned from the high stress, part-time job I'd been doing for the last three years: managing a couple of multimillion dollar government contracts for a firm in Washington, D.C. Then, I packed my bags and stepped off to train to become a yoga teacher.

Total immersion is a wonderful way to transform old habits! During my training, I lost about eight pounds and most of my back pain *and* gained a whole new outlook on life. I also made new friends who were treading the same path toward better health and wellness. It's much easier to walk that new path when someone else is walking beside you, sharing your journey. I later came to realize that one of the best parts of my yoga training was my involvement with my fellow students. In my class of 30, there were people of all cultures, sizes and ages. We learned how to modify and replace certain exercises with alternatives so that everyone could participate, and that was, as the TV commercial states, "priceless."

When my training was finished, I started teaching a couple of classes a week at the hospital wellness center. Before you could say, "supercalifragilisticexpialidocious," my wonderful mentor decided that it would be great if the hospital could offer Pilates classes as well. Off I went to become trained as a Pilates instructor. I love Pilates. As a young girl, I had danced and was pretty good at it. I discovered that Joseph

Pilates began his teaching in New York by helping dancers from the New York City Ballet. There was even an old 8mm film of him as a young man teaching dancers at a Jacob's Pillow Dance Festival in the Berkshires of Massachusetts. I especially loved watching that film since I grew up in the Berkshires and had received a scholarship to summer training at Jacob's Pillow when I was 12!

The Pilates training I received at The Body College in Washington, D.C., was fabulous. However, as part of the certification process, I also needed to complete 20 classes with a certified instructor, and that was very different from my yoga training. These classes were taught by a young woman in her early twenties who had never been pregnant, had no idea what a hot flash was, and who insisted that when you do an abdominal crunch, you should be able to pull your belly in—it should not pooch out (like mine did). Well, since that time, I've seen many other young women teaching Pilates who believe the same thing (give them about 20 years and see if they don't change their tune...). I've also met lots of older women who think they can't do Pilates because it's too difficult, or it's their daughter's exercise program, not theirs. I'm happy to tell you that those who have come to my classes have lost inches, reduced their pain, and gained confidence, flexibility and, in some cases, bone mass. They are absolutely able to do the exercises with my modifications, and they now love Pilates! Everything is possible if you believe!

Before long, I was teaching more and more classes a week and becoming more and more fit. For a couple of years, I taught 12 classes a week of either yoga or Pilates! All the while, I continued my learning and earned certificates in somatics, acu-yoga (which uses acupressure in combination with yoga poses), healing touch, ancient ayurvedic physical healing—and the list goes on. I absolutely love my new career. I have no back pain, have lowered my blood pressure to normal so that I no longer need medication, and am healthier and more fit now than I was at age 20. I'm passionate about helping others achieve similar results.

In my classes, I always gave so much information about exercises that specifically help alleviate pain in the neck, hips and back, etc., that eventually, students began to come in early or stay late to ask what they could do for their hip or back pain, neck and shoulder pain, leg pain, etc. I would give them the exercises that I knew firsthand would help, and the next week they would tell everyone in the class how great they felt. My reputation grew and grew.

Now that I'd found my adventurous, creative thinking inner self, I realized that *this* was my purpose in life: Teaching others how to use simple exercises and techniques that make it possible to live pain free again! My AHA! moment arrived with the recognition of my gift for knowing the right relaxation technique or the perfect exercise to help someone end pain. I'm happiest when sharing this information with others.

I knew I needed to get the word out to as many people as possible, so I developed my own program called *Get Rid of Sciatic Pain for Good!* I first presented this program as a workshop, and it was very successful, so I recorded a video demonstrating the three best exercises and began marketing that DVD on Amazon and other places. It soon became my best-selling product and still is to this day.

I love to spread the word about healing chronic back pain, because I know how much this information is needed. If you think about it, I'm sure you know at least a couple of people who often complain about their sore backs, or who have missed work due to back pain, or who take prescription drugs to relieve their pain. I'll bet everyone reading this book right now has felt nagging back or neck pain at some point!

It never ceases to amaze me how many of us have back issues! According to the American Chiropractic Association, 70 to 85 percent of Americans suffer from back pain at some time in their lives, and as we age, back pain becomes increasingly likely. Wow!

In fact, here are a few more interesting facts about back pain from The American Chiropractic Association:

Low back pain is the fifth most common reason for all physician visits in the United States.[1,2]

Back pain is the most frequent cause of activity limitation in people younger than 45 years old.[3]

Approximately one quarter of U.S. adults reported having low back pain lasting at least one whole day in the past three months, and 7.6 percent reported at least one episode of severe acute low back pain within a one-year period.[4]

One-half of all working Americans admit to having back pain symptoms each year.[5]

Approximately 2 percent of the U.S. work force is compensated for back injuries each year.[6]

Americans spend at least $50 billion per year on back pain—and that's just for the more easily identified costs.[7]

Many chronic back pain sufferers believe that invasive surgery is their only option, or that they are out of options and just have to learn to live with the pain. This book is all about the *many* therapies and techniques that are available all over the world today to heal your back pain. No one should have to live with chronic pain.

Doctors who practice traditional Western medicine are trained to treat a physical symptom. They believe that if you have a backache, you need some pain medication and ice. If the pain worsens, they take your blood pressure, maybe draw some blood and run tests, or weigh you, but their assessment usually does not include looking at the way you walk or how you are sitting in the chair in front of them. They rarely ask about the stress in your life.

In contrast, all of the practitioners and therapists that I interviewed for this book actively treat the whole person. They recognize that if you are having major stress in your life, it may be, literally, giving you a pain in the neck. What you may really need then, are some stress management techniques along with your back exercises in order prevent a reoccurrence.

I'm here to tell you that not only is it possible to relax all of the muscles in your back without medication, or expensive equipment, but that you can feel *so* much better in as little as five minutes! Every time I use a technique featured in this book, I say to myself, "Everyone who suffers from chronic back pain needs to know about this!" In the last several years, I have shown thousands how to use this program, and every time I show them even one technique that can make a huge difference, they have an OMG moment: Their pain is relieved and they feel better.

I have helped thousands of people relieve their chronic back pain through my "Three-Step Approach" which consists of relaxation first, then stretching, then strengthening. My assessment does include asking personal questions about stress and lifestyle issues. Sometimes, I'll even go to a client's workplace and see how his or her desk is set up. I then offer advice on adjusting chair height or using a footstool, or even taking breaks every hour to stretch the lower back. I know that if you get to the bottom of your symptoms, you can heal the pain.

I've seen many people helped by all of the therapies mentioned in this book, because these also treat your entire self—mind, body and spirit. So take heart—you *can* relieve your back pain. And the best part is that it may be much easier than you think!

My dream is that all of you who are suffering from back pain right now will find your personal best solution within these pages. Every**body** is different and what works for me may not work for you, or vice versa. The point is that there are plenty of options—don't give up simply because the one method you've tried didn't work. *You don't have to live with the pain.*

My mission in life is to use my creativity, enthusiasm and humor to help people take charge of their own health and well-being and to age well with joy and laughter. I want to help you feel better!

Now you know a little bit about me, and how I resolved my own sciatic nerve pain, let's get right into the "meat" of this book. Enjoy *STOP Back Pain* and your own new lease on life!

Best of health—especially back health—to you all,

Kathi

Chapter One

The Many Causes of Back, Neck and Sciatic Nerve Pain

"The aim of the wise is not to secure pleasure, but to avoid pain."

—Aristotle

Did you know that your sciatic nerve is actually several nerve cords that exit through your tailbone, travelling through your deep buttocks muscles and then down the back of your legs? On this route through your body, these nerve cords pass through the rough territory of some pretty thick muscles, such as your piriformis and hamstrings. When these muscles become inflamed or tight and inflexible, they can press on the sciatic nerve, causing you pain. Sometimes, the pain is barely noticeable, but many times it is excruciating pain that travels from your hip to your toes. I refer to sciatic nerve pain throughout this book because this nerve is such a long one and it affects so much of your back, hips and legs, that simply using the term *back pain* doesn't begin to describe the territory of sciatic nerve pain.

When tight or inflamed muscles are the cause of your back, neck or sciatic nerve pain, relief can be found relatively quickly through specific relaxation techniques and simple exercises. However, if you don't make these exercise routines a part of your daily life, pain will become another unwelcome frequent visitor—like your mother-in-law who asks when you're going to do something with your hair every time she sees you. ☺

Many believe that a **herniated disk** is the only cause of back, neck or sciatic nerve pain; however, there are many other causes. *Disks* are the small, sponge-like cushions between our vertebrae that function like the shock absorbers in our cars; *herniated disks* are disks that have worn out. Just like with our car, the wear and tear of age and injury can cause disks to flatten out and bulge or even "rupture," which means they tear open and some of the gel-like substance inside pushes outward, putting pressure on the nerves in the spine.

People with **piriformis syndrome** can experience severe sciatic nerve pain. In this case, the piriformis muscle becomes so tight that it forgets how to relax. (Having a tight butt is not always a good thing!) This thick muscle runs across your buttocks from hip to tailbone. It travels a path right through your hip bone. When it's tense and tight all the time, it's constantly pulling your hip toward your tailbone or vice versa, throwing your whole pelvic region out of balance. You can imagine how this can cause pressure on your sciatic nerve and the excruciating pain that follows. While I'm not Harry Potter, and can't wave a magic wand and mutter a charm to make it go away, I can teach you a very simple way to massage that muscle to relax it, and then some fantastic stretches that you'll need to do every day to keep the muscle from tensing all the time. When you do these exercises regularly, you will find relief that's better than Harry's pumpkin juice or butter beer!

Another culprit that causes a lot of grief for those who do lots of crunches or who are proponents of the "feast, then famine" method of abdominal exercise is the **iliopsoas** muscle. This one is on the front of your body and it travels from the front side of your vertebrae to the front of your hip joint.

The iliopsoas also can get too tight, *and* it's more difficult to relax and stretch than your hamstrings or piriformis are because it's located deep in your pelvic region. There is hope, however, and you'll find relief in the chapters that follow.

Sometimes, a form of **arthritis** called *stenosis* can cause either neck or sciatic nerve pain due to a painful narrowing of your spinal canal. This narrowing causes pressure on your spinal cord or several spinal nerves. And this dirty rotten scoundrel can occur in either your neck or your lower back—yikes!

Strains, sprains and spasms can occur when you lift something heavy like that bag of garden soil or too many weights at the gym, or you shovel snow after a big storm. Any and all of these can cause inflammation and swelling which, in turn, cause pressure on any or all of the spinal nerves and the resulting nasty pain.

Traumatic injury like a car accident can also damage the spine and cause swelling and pressure on the nerves of your spine. An additional problem that often occurs after an injury such as an auto accident or fall from a horse, etc., is the "haunting effect." This is when the pain comes back again and again long after your doctor has released you from treatment. Most often, this continual haunting occurs because of your natural body language, which tells the left side of your body to favor the right until it heals (or vice versa). After a period of time, the wiring between your brain and the non-damaged side of your body becomes mixed up and your muscles forget how to completely relax. *Somatics* is a modality that retrains your body to make those connections work properly again, enabling you to completely relax so that your body can heal and the pain can leave—and never come back!

Save your **sacroiliac**! Inflammation of the sacroiliac joint is believed to be caused by an abnormal movement of the joint. As a teenager, my sister fell down the stairs and injured her sacroiliac (ouch!), which then gave her problems for years. When the sacroiliac joint becomes inflamed, the portion of the sciatic nerve that runs directly in front of the joint can be irritated, causing sciatic nerve pain. Range of motion exercises designed specifically for the sacroiliac joint usually restore normal movement and alleviate the irritation of your sciatic nerve.

Osteoporosis can also cause sciatic nerve pain. As we age, we can lose mass or density from our bones, making them porous and brittle. This is called *osteoporosis*. When you have osteoporosis, simple daily chores such as lifting a laundry basket can cause the front part of the weak bones to fracture, giving you a real "pain the backside." Most often, the first place osteoporosis shows up is in the hips and lower back. It is possible with exercise and supplements to restore some bone mass or density naturally and I'll cover that in the chapters that follow.

Other conditions such as tumors, infections and disease can cause back, neck or sciatic nerve pain, which is why your most important first step when back pain strikes is to get a diagnosis from your doctor. Certainly, you would want a tumor or infection taken care of quickly. You can regain your strength later, but first you must heal the underlying disease. With so many causes for back pain, I can't stress enough the importance of seeing your doctor first before starting any exercise or strengthening program.

Chapter Two

Symptoms You Wouldn't Wish on Your Worst Enemy!

"One good thing about music, when it hits you, you feel no pain."

—Bob Marley

I've heard several different descriptions of back pain and sciatic nerve pain and have come to the conclusion that while the pain is different for everyone depending on the cause, there are many similarities as well.

Pain can vary widely, from a mild ache to a sharp, burning sensation, or excruciating discomfort. I love the word *excruciating*. I think it perfectly describes the most horrible pain. It's like the curse that my favorite little wizard Harry Potter learns: "Crucio!" which tortures an opponent unmercifully. Sometimes, the pain feels like a jolt or electric shock. It may be worse when you cough or sneeze, and sitting for long periods will aggravate your symptoms. Back pain usually affects only one side, but don't be fooled: Many people, including yours truly, have worked it out of one side of the body only to have it show up on the other side a couple of weeks later! Experience is a great teacher. This is why I *always* recommend working both sides of your body for optimum results.

Pain that radiates from your lower back through one buttock, and down the back of your leg, is the most common description of sciatic nerve pain. You may feel pain almost anywhere along the highway that your spinal and sciatic nerves follow, but it's more likely to follow the path from your lower back to your heels.

Sometimes symptoms also include:

Numbness or muscle weakness along the nerve pathway in your leg or foot. In some cases, you can even feel pain in one part of your leg or foot and numbness in another.
That pins-and-needles feeling, or tingling like when your leg falls asleep. You may feel this in your leg, toes or foot.
Pain or cramping in your legs after standing for a long period of time, or when you walk.

Sometimes, people feel only hip or knee pain and are not aware that it can be sciatic nerve pain.

Some may find it impossible to walk, sit or even lie down without pain; this was the case with an uncle of mine.

My own sciatic nerve pain usually shows up as a pain in my butt—literally. After a long road trip, or sitting at my desk for several hours, I'll feel pain radiating from my butt to my lower back and back to my hip and buttocks. Not fun! I now know exactly what to do to relieve it and keep it from ruining my trip, though, and that makes life *much* easier!

Whatever your symptoms are, trust that there is hope. You can end your chronic back, neck and sciatic nerve pain and keep it from coming back. There are many options for treatment, as you'll see.

Chapter Three

Types of Treatments

"All parts of the body which have a function if used in moderation and exercised in labors in which each is accustomed, become thereby healthy, well developed and age more slowly, but if unused they become liable to disease, defective in growth and age quickly."

—Hippocrates

Several types of treatments for back pain are available. You might find one particularly helpful, or a combination of treatments might be best for you.

Physical Therapy

Physical therapy, or PT, is covered by most medical insurance and works very well to relax your muscles and relieve your pain. Your therapist will also teach you several exercises that strengthen your neck or back, which you should continue at home after your pain is gone. Especially if you have a herniated disk, your physical therapist will design a program of exercises to help prevent reoccurrences.

Physical therapy will include exercises to help correct your posture, adjust your gait if necessary, and strengthen all of the muscles that support your neck or back and improve your flexibility. Although it may seem counterintuitive, your doctor will most likely recommend that you start physical therapy, exercise or both as early as possible for the best results. The days of lying around waiting for your back to "heal" are long gone. Doctors everywhere now agree that the best results are achieved through movement and exercise.

I will add that relaxation is the key to regaining your strength and flexibility so don't skip this part. I'm talking to all of you type A personalities out there! Your busy, nonstop mind may not like to spend five minutes relaxing those back muscles, but *your back* will most definitely say thank you!

Tom Papke, a physical therapist that I interviewed, says that "a PT assessment starts when you greet your patient in the waiting room—how does the person sit, stand up, walk to the examination room—and continues until you get to know that person almost as well as you know yourself." This type of close observation enables the PT to understand where the symptoms are coming from and how to help you heal completely. Tom treats the whole person—the only way to truly heal the pain. "You can't just hand everyone a sheet of exercises as a sort of 'one size fits all.'" I agree wholeheartedly with Tom.

Medication

Medication is another treatment that is usually covered by insurance. There are over–the-counter and prescription drugs that can relax your muscles, reduce inflammation and calm your spasms. These offer temporary results that may eliminate your pain, but they do not resolve the underlying problem. So, while they may be needed at the beginning to keep you sane, you really have to examine the underlying cause of your back, neck or sciatic nerve pain and decide on a plan for treatment that gets to the heart of the matter. That way, you can keep that pain from returning again and again.

I will say a word here about a supplement that I recommend to reduce inflammation. Omega-3s, an essential fatty acid, have a great track record for reducing and preventing inflammation, so if you're not currently taking a daily omega-3 supplement, try adding one.

Herbal Remedies

Herbal remedies such as willow bark have also been quite effective in reducing pain and swelling. Devil's claw is another herbal treatment used for pain relief, and bromelain (pineapple extract) is another of Mother Nature's powerful anti-inflammatories. Some studies have found that a plaster made from cayenne pepper applied directly to skin works as well as pain patches or gels do. The capsaicin in cayenne interferes with our pain receptors, sort of like novocaine does. Personally, I have not tried the cayenne pepper. I can't bring myself to rub hot stuff on my skin. If it makes my mouth feel like it's on fire...

Epidural Steroid Injections

Epidural steroid injections are often recommended by doctors because they yield quick results—especially if you are in so much pain that you can't function. These corticosteroids are useful for stopping and preventing inflammation around your irritated nerves, helping to relieve your pain, but their effect is often minimal or nonexistent, and any positive effect you feel is short term. In addition, there are many side effects to corticosteroids, so doctors will only prescribe this treatment a limited number of times. I've known many people who got some relief the first time they tried an epidural steroid shot and thought it was the answer to their prayers, but when the injection was repeated a second time, they felt no relief at all. Disappointment set in like the fog over London.

Chiropractic

Chiropractic adjustment, which is also called spinal manipulation, provides relief for many people. In fact, several studies have shown chiropractic adjustment to be as effective as any other treatment for relieving back or neck pain. The manipulation or adjustment involves moving a joint beyond its usual range of motion, but not beyond the range of motion the joint is designed to experience, which is why you sometimes hear a cracking noise during your chiropractic adjustment. Since motion is the best way to increase blood flow and free up tension in the back, chiropractic adjustment can relieve pain quickly, thus improving your body's physical function.

In fact, you might be surprised to know that originally, chiropractic manipulation was designed to treat many illnesses in the body, such as hearing loss and immune disorders. During the influenza (flu) epidemic of 1918 in the United States, influenza patients who received chiropractic care experienced fantastic results while those under medical care died like flies. According to Dan Murphy, DC, "Reports show that in New York City, during the influenza epidemic of 1918, out of every 10,000 cases medically treated, 950 died. These figures are exact, for in that city these are reportable diseases. In the same epidemic, under drugless methods (chiropractic), only 25 patients died of influenza out of every 10,000 cases." Wow! Gimme some of that spinal manipulation!

Chiropractic manipulation is performed by a chiropractic doctor, or an osteopathic doctor.

Massage

Massage therapy is good for the body *and* good for the soul! Many people find massage helpful in treating back, neck or sciatic nerve pain because massage relaxes the muscles and brings good blood flow to the area. When your muscles are relaxed, they don't put as much pressure on your nerves, so pain is reduced. However, be sure to use a certified massage therapist to avoid having an untrained person cause further damage.

Again, with massage, pain relief may be temporary as it does not address the root of the problem, unless stress is your main issue and you receive a weekly massage to release all those extra stress hormones coursing through your body. Massage certainly feels better than some other options do and works at least as well as medication does. One of my goals for this year is to have therapeutic massage twice a month. I just feel sooooooo good afterward, and that sense of well-being stays with me for several days.

Acupuncture

Acupuncture has been proven very effective in treating chronic pain. In a 2009 study published in the *Archives of Internal Medicine,* acupuncture was shown to be more effective at relieving back pain than medication.

Many people are afraid to try acupuncture because it involves needles. I've had acupuncture several times and usually I don't even feel the needles going into my body. They are thinner than a horse's hair, and the acupuncturist snaps them into the specific vital points in your body based upon your diagnosis. You then get to lie quietly and rest for several minutes. Many people even fall asleep during acupuncture because it's so relaxing. After several minutes, your acupuncturist will come back and adjust the needles. Mostly, this means that she or he will twist them. Once in a while, I will feel a little tingling when this twisting is done, but no pain. Many insurance companies now also cover at least part of this treatment, so it's worth looking into.

Acupuncture is one of the many therapies that work on the subtle energy of the body—the vital energy that is both inside *and* outside of your body. This energy follows pathways called meridians and is released from the body through energy centers called chakras. How the energy flows affects your organs, glands, and other areas of the body. Based upon a thorough diagnosis, your acupuncturist will insert needles into specific points along the meridians to relieve your pain and get your energy flowing smoothly again.

Acupressure

Acupressure works on the same principles as acupuncture, but without the needles. I know a few people who are so afraid of needles that they see an acupressure therapist instead of an acupuncturist, and they experience good results, so here is another option for those with needle phobia. In acupressure, the therapist uses light finger pressure on the vital points instead of needles.

Reflexology

Reflexology is another therapy that is becoming very popular in the United States and treats the whole person. In reflexology, as in massage, the practitioner places pressure on your feet or hands, but in a certain pattern that eliminates pain or energy blocks in the rest of your body. Hundreds of reflexology studies from many countries have shown that reflexology is effective at treating a variety of physical complaints including back pain. The premise of this therapy is that certain reflexes located in your feet and hands can be activated with light finger or thumb pressure to release energy blockages.

Audrey Herrick, my niece, who practices both reflexology and Reiki (a form of mind/body medicine that will be discussed later), explains: "Many people prefer reflexology as a way to release the pain in their neck or back because the only part of the body that's worked on is the feet or hands. The painful area is not touched at all, yet receives the benefit of pain release." I have sampled her reflexology on several occasions and she truly is a gifted healer. And I know that some of you are thinking this is "hocus-pocus," but I can tell you that thousands of people that I know have found tremendous relief from Reflexology. Give it a try, you may love it!

Mind/Body Medicine

Mind/body medicine is gaining in popularity in the west, thanks to pioneers like Dr. Deepak Chopra, Dr. Joan Borysenko, Dr. Darren Weissman and Dr. Carolyn Dean. These masters are among the leaders bringing attention to natural healing methods that include proper nutrition, the healing of emotional wounds, and the examination of how our thoughts affect our health.

Many mind/body techniques have been studied by Western science and proven effective in treating back or neck pain. Here are a few that I know for sure work, as I've gotten relief from them myself.

Emotional Freedom Technique (EFT or tapping)

Emotional Freedom Technique works on the same principle as acupuncture only gentle tapping is used on specific vital points while you repeat a personalized phrase. The phrase is changed as you tap different points and you repeat the pattern of tapping three or more times. This takes less than three minutes to do and is very easy to learn. This treatment is also currently being used with much success in treating veterans with post traumatic stress disorder.[8] Yay for EFT!

The Lifeline Technique

Dr. Darren Weissman calls his healing therapy "The Lifeline Technique." Basically, this technique uses the subtle energy of the body and the power of the mind to treat core imbalances that bring on symptoms. According to Dr. Weissman, our conscious mind would never "choose" to be in pain; therefore, it's our subconscious mind that is giving us grief. And, if we uncover the emotions that we are internalizing, denying, or disconnecting from, then we can heal the symptoms. Darren has devised a system that incorporates muscle testing, powerful affirmations, visualization and other methods to identify the real cause of pain. He believes that only when the root causes are identified can the pain be relieved. Infinite love and gratitude to Dr. Darren!

The Sedona Method

"The Sedona Method" is another process of using the power of our minds to let go of symptoms, fears and anxiety. Hale Dwoskin, author of *The Sedona Method,* explains that the body is able to self-heal and, if we get out of its way, the body can heal addictions, depression, insomnia and more. I have been fortunate enough to witness Hale use this method to help a baby boomer who was suffering from chronic, severe headaches and neck pain, and for a few seconds this man felt no pain! It's easy to see that with extended use, the Sedona Method could heal his pain completely. Hail, Hale!

The Mindbody Prescription

No book on healing back pain would be complete without mentioning the significant body of work done by the great "Western pioneer" Dr. John Sarno (he is trained in Western medicine *and* is a pioneer in treating back pain!). Dr. Sarno has healed thousands of people's back pain with his "Mindbody Prescription." Like the others mentioned previously, Dr. Sarno works with underlying repressed emotions to get to the root of the problem. He presents specific scientific evidence showing that the brain creates physical symptoms and can also alleviate them. As a Western trained physician, Dr. Sarno bases his Mindbody Prescription on scientific principles that many physicians can understand and use to treat patients with back pain. In my opinion, Dr. Sarno's books should be required reading in all medical schools.

There are many more mind/body techniques that I've no personal knowledge of yet, but as I discover them, I'll keep you posted!

Surgery

Surgery has become the treatment of last resort. Only when a compressed nerve causes incontinence or significant weakness, or when you have pain that gets progressively worse or doesn't improve with other therapies, will surgery be recommended.

Surgical options include diskectomy and microdiskectomy. In diskectomy, surgeons remove a portion of a herniated disk that's pressing on a nerve. Ideally, most of the disk is left intact to preserve as much of the normal anatomy as possible. Sometimes, a surgeon will perform this operation through a small incision while looking through a microscope. Don't you just love modern technology?

Success rates for standard diskectomy and microdiskectomy are about the same, which is only about 50 percent success. You may have less pain and recover more quickly with microdiskectomy, due to smaller incisions but, as with any surgery, the risks are high. Our spines are very complicated and intricate, with more nerves running through them than tea grown in China! Some risks associated with surgery are infection, a tear in the membrane that covers the spinal cord, a blood clot in a leg vein and neurological deterioration. Going under the knife in this case truly is a desperate measure.

What if you need instant topical relief? There are products and home remedies that provide what you're looking for, but as you'll see, some work better than others.

Chapter Four

Pain Creams, Patches, Heating Pads—Oh My!

"Pain is deeper than all thought; laughter is higher than all pain."

—Elbert Hubbard

Ice for the Pain

To ice or not to ice: that is the question that William Shakespeare originally asked. He changed it afterwards because he didn't want the director or the studio to know that he had back issues and file a lawsuit against him. ☺ In fact, another of his most quoted lines was: "The first thing we should do is kill all the lawyers!" (No offense intended...)

Anyway, back to the most common question people ask about back pain: Is it better to ice or heat the area? Let's take a look at reasons behind each procedure, and maybe things will become clearer.

When the piriformis muscle starts to spasm, the body begins to send more white blood cells and fewer red blood cells to the butt. This is how the immune system takes care of the injury. The problem is that the red blood cells bring oxygen to the muscles and when the muscle is in spasm, it needs oxygen for healing! Secondly, the brain gets the signal for feeling pain in the butt. The butt muscles automatically contract, restricting the blood flow even more, essentially making that "pain in the butt" worse! Heat increases the blood flow to the area, bringing much needed oxygen, which helps heal the piriformis muscle. Heat also relaxes the muscle, reducing the pain. Plus, it just feels good.

Heat is *not* recommended for sprains or strains, however, due to the swelling that occurs with these injuries. Swelling from sprains or strains should be reduced first, and cold does that best. Essentially, cold constricts the walls of blood vessels, reducing swelling. Cold also numbs the nerve endings, numbing out the pain.

Most doctors recommend ice for the first 24 to 48 hours after an injury, sprain or strain. It's important to start icing right away to relieve the swelling, so if you don't have an ice pack available, grab a bag of ice or frozen veggies and get right on it!

Once the swelling begins to go down, it's important to exercise the back muscles to get them healthy and strong as soon as possible. Most people feel better when they use heat before and after exercise. A word of caution: Heat is not recommended for inflamed muscles as the heat can worsen the inflammation. Another reason to use ice!

There are many ways to get ice to your sore muscles. As for what method of icing to use, recent studies have shown that ice chips mixed with a little bit of cold water in a self-sealing plastic bag works best.[9] To prevent leakage, wrap a hand towel around your homemade ice pack. If you are unable to make your own ice pack, the frozen gel packs are a good second choice, but try to stay away from the ones that contain chemicals. When my kids were younger, I witnessed a couple of high school athletes use those and receive a nasty chemical burn when they leaked—the burn was worse than the original injury!

A "fisherman's ice blanket" works really well to get a large portion of your back iced all at the same time. It's a small plastic blanket with pockets of gel that fishermen use to cover the freshly caught fish in their coolers; you can find it in an outdoor sports equipment store. The blanket can be rolled up so it doesn't take up much space in your freezer. When you need it, simply unroll it and lie down on it. I wrap a blanket or a beach towel over the fisherman's ice blanket as well, just to be safe.

Recent studies have also shown that ten minutes on and twenty minutes off works best for reducing swelling. The recommended time used to be twenty minutes on and twenty minutes off but I could never stand to have an ice pack on for more than ten minutes, so I'm glad they've changed those recommendations!

When Heat Helps

Applying heat to a painful area is used when the condition is chronic because heat loosens up tissues and improves blood flow to the area. Most doctors recommend moist heat because dry heat tends to dry out your skin too much, so toss out your old heating pad—especially if you tend to use it at bedtime and fall asleep with it (not a good practice!). An inexpensive way to get moist heat to your lower back is to toss a wet towel in the microwave for a few seconds. Be careful not to get the towel too hot or you may cause a burn. When you've tested it and it feels the right temperature, wrap it around yourself or lie down on it.

Hot tubs are also a good method for getting moist heat to your back. So is a hot shower.

Patches, Gels and Creams

Personally, I don't like the smell of the patches, gels or creams; however, I have tested a few and they do work to reduce the pain. The camphor and menthol work as a team to lessen the sensitivity of heat receptors in the sore areas and activate the cold receptors, relieving your pain.

Salonpas® is one patch that I've tested and written about in my blog. My son and I both found that this patch worked well to relieve the pain for several hours. Salonpas® is also approved by the FDA. Several other patches that we tried did very little or nothing for the pain, yet still smelled bad.

Gels and creams like Bengay and IcyHot not only smell bad, but are greasy and can stain some types of clothing, so I don't personally recommend them.

* * *

Next, we'll look at some treatments you may not have heard of or considered, and why they work well alone or in combination with other treatments.

Chapter Five

The East West Connection

"You treat a disease, you win, you lose. You treat a person, I guarantee you, you'll win, no matter what the outcome."

—Patch Adams, MD.

I've witnessed women use Pilates or yoga to address their bone loss, and they've gained back most of what they had lost. Others have completely healed their back, neck or sciatic nerve pain through the exercises I teach based on **yoga, somatics, Pilates or acupressure**. Again, every*body* is different and you must research the best choice for you. Thank goodness there are so many choices!

That said, I find it funny when I hear people say that they are going for "traditional" medical treatment, and they mean Western medicine, instead of what they refer to as "alternative" or Eastern medicine. By definition, the word traditional means "inherited or customary thought," and "the handing down of information, beliefs and customs by word of mouth or written word." The problem is semantics, I suppose. Eastern medicine is the actual traditional method. Much of what we think of as Western medicine has been around for a very short time. My own belief is that the two types of medicine should always work hand in hand. Modern technology cannot be ignored. There is much that Western medicine has taught us about out physical bodies and our minds through recent technological advances such as MRIs, ultrasound, thermography and blood screenings.

What follows is some information about several Eastern medical treatments, all of which are preventative and are effective for healing back pain but are usually not covered by medical insurance. My hope is that very soon insurance companies will see that prevention is much less costly than surgery, medication and hospital stays, and will cover Eastern treatments, Western treatments, and mind/body techniques.

Qigong

I have practiced qigong (chee-gong), a practice similar to tai chi, but even more ancient, and find it enjoyable as well as healing. Both tai chi and qigong have been proven by Western scientific research to be very effective for improving immune function, lowering blood pressure and heart disease risk, and reducing anxiety.[10,11]

These ancient Chinese traditional medicines have been in use for thousands of years. I enjoy the slow motion movements of qigong and the meditative aspect. Qigong's use of breathing patterns while exercising is very similar to yoga, which you already know I love! While there is little scientific evidence that qigong can help strengthen your back, I have seen many people use it to improve their overall health and strength, and improve posture, breathing and stamina—all of which help the back to heal and can prevent recurrences of neck, back or sciatic nerve pain. Currently, the Mayo Clinic is sponsoring studies of qigong master Chunyi Lin's work that he calls "Spring Forest Qigong." His healing practices have helped many people not only stop their pain, but also heal tumors and chronic diseases, so I expect that western science will be catching up with this ancient medicine soon!

Ayurveda

Ayurveda is the world's most ancient medicine. It originated in India and evolved there over thousands of years. The term *ayurveda* is a combination of the Sanskrit words *ayur,* which means "life," and *veda* which means "science." The translation, then, is "the science of life."

Ayurveda is still the most widely practiced form of medicine in India today and there are medical schools there where you can train to be an ayurvedic physician. Deepak Chopra is both an ayurvedic physician and a Western medical doctor. Recently, ayurvedic hospitals have been set up in Japan and Germany, and there is a college of ayurvedic medicine in the U.S. that trains ayurvedic physicians.

One of the basic beliefs in ayurveda is that our health can be perfect if our mind and body are in harmony and our interaction with the entire universe is natural and wholesome. (Ayurveda is the original mind/body medicine.) According to ayurveda, disease arises when a person is "not at ease" with the universe. These disruptions to our natural harmony can be physical, emotional, spiritual or a combination of all three.

Ayurvedic treatments are based upon your "dosha" or life energies: pitta, kapha, and vata. For instance, I'm sure that you know someone who loves hot sauce—the hotter the better—and someone else who can't stand even a little bit of it. If you look at the doshas of these two people, you will most likely find that one primarily has a pitta dosha: Spicy food upsets his whole constitution. The other person has a kapha dosha and needs hot foods to balance his constitution. It all makes sense when you understand how it works—this is just one example so that you can get the idea. It is believed that each of us falls into one of three doshas, or categories, and the treatments are based upon a person's primary dosha. (We all have a little bit of all three, but usually one is more prominent.)

For treatment of neck or back pain, your ayurvedic practitioner would first want you to cleanse your body of impurities, both inside and out. After your cleanse, you may be prescribed some herbal remedies, ayurvedic massage or yoga exercises.

Healing Touch and Reiki

Healing touch and Reiki have become much more widely used in the West as well. Both of these techniques adjust the body's subtle energy to help the healing process. Practitioners balance the meridians and chakras, just as with acupuncture, except that instead of using needles, practitioners use their hands to remove energy blocks and restore balance. Again, meridians are the energy pathways of the body; chakras are specific energy vortexes in our bodies that influence all areas of the body. All of the meridians run through the vital energy centers called chakras. Blockages of the energy flowing through the meridians and chakras can also affect our emotions and mental state.

I have experienced both techniques and highly recommend them. As a healing touch practitioner myself, I have seen many people find relief from back or neck and shoulder pain as a result of using this amazing energy medicine.

In recent years, several traditional Eastern medicines have become more widely accepted and used in the West—acupuncture, herbal remedies and therapeutic massage are the top three. Many health insurance companies now pay for acupuncture, and some offer discounts or partial reimbursement for therapeutic massage, yoga, and qigong classes. There are even a few hospitals in Florida that require healing touch therapy before and after surgery, because they have discovered that patients heal much faster with far fewer complications when healing touch is provided. Renowned cardiac surgeon Dr. Mehmet Oz now recommends Reiki for his patients undergoing heart surgery because he has discovered that when patients have Reiki before and after surgery, they experience fewer blood clots, which are a big problem with this type of surgery, and their recuperation time is shorter.

My own experience has taught me that what works for one person does not necessarily work for another. We are all unique—no two people are exactly alike. Therefore, each of us needs to find our healthy balance in our own way. In many instances, it's a combination of therapies that works best.

When you are in excruciating pain, it's essential for your sanity that you get immediate relief from the pain before you begin a program of repair and prevention. Chronic back or neck pain can have a negative impact on your life. Often, it brings with it anxiety and depression. It can affect your ability to work, sleep and perform other daily activities. Recent studies have shown that chronic pain lasting longer than six months can cause cognitive decline.[12] When we suffer chronic pain, we actually lose grey matter in our brains. Therefore, stopping the pain is your first step.

Most of us still turn to Western pharmacology for pain relief; however, the evidence is strong that techniques associated with Eastern traditions—such as yoga, massage and qigong—work well as a second step toward recovering strength and flexibility, and preventing back, neck, and sciatic nerve pain from returning. I recommend trying a little of each technique until you find the combination that works best for you, and then stick to it like glue!

Chapter Six

Stress and Your Back or Neck Pain

"Never underestimate the power of your emotions..."

—Unknown

I know many people who, without even realizing it, send all of their stress straight to their necks or lower backs. After a few weeks or months of holding on to stress in your back, or carrying that "stress backpack" in your neck and shoulders, it only takes getting out of bed in the morning or reaching over to pick up your socks to bring on a full blown episode of sciatic nerve pain.

In today's fast-paced world, it's difficult to keep up with all that we have to do for ourselves and others. My own children tease me about my cell phone, which they think is an antique. It's only two years old! I have a nephew in the fourth grade who is learning what I did in high school. The world is changing so fast that sometimes it makes my head spin. It also makes for a lot of stress and is causing a lot of stress-related illness, including chronic back pain.

You might wonder why stress has become an increasing problem in recent years. Well, Bill Joy, chief scientist at Sun Microsystems, has an interesting theory. Bill estimates that the speed of change is doubling exponentially every 18 months. And according to him, the speed of change will only increase in coming months, years and decades. Change is stressful, even good change. Think about getting married or having a baby—these are examples of good changes in our lives, yet they can certainly be stressful!

The problem today is that many people are constantly stressed out. In a chronic stress condition, your body continually releases stress hormones such as cortisol and adrenaline. They've gotten a bad reputation in recent years, but these stress hormones serve a valid purpose. Cortisol's job in our body is to take glucose away from our other bodily systems and functions, and get it to our leg muscles quickly, so that we can run away very quickly from a ferocious animal on the prowl. That was very useful back in the day when a ferocious wild animal was the only danger we regularly faced—although I know many people who refer to their boss as a ferocious animal…. Another stress hormone, called adrenaline, increases our heart rate and elevates blood pressure so we have the stamina to run away quickly. Cortisol slows down bodily functions that would be nonessential in a "fight or flight" situation, such as running away from a grizzly bear. It suppresses the immune system and the digestive process; slows the reproductive system; and affects mood, motivation and fear.

Currently, we find ourselves "stressing out" about losing our jobs or homes, or worrying about how on earth we are going to help our kids pay for college with tuition costs rising higher than Mt. Everest. Many are working in jobs that they don't even like, but feel stuck there for financial or other reasons, and the stress is literally killing them. Maybe you have the "boss from hell," and you're on edge all the time, wondering when the next explosion will hit and who will be blown apart by the verbal mortars.

All of this constant worrying triggers the release of stress hormones way too often, so that too much cortisol and adrenaline spin around the racetrack of the bloodstream, causing a big traffic jam! As a result, our immune and digestive systems, and even, sometimes, our brains, are deprived of glucose, a much needed fuel. After a while, these systems, and our brain cells, begin to deteriorate—sort of like that tiny rust spot on the side of your car that turns into a huge hole in a matter of weeks. This is how organs and glands become diseased. *You* are no longer at ease, and so your body becomes "dis-eased."

In fact, according to a 20 year study by Kaiser Permanente, 70 to 85 percent of all illnesses sending patients to their doctors were caused by stress—not just aggravated by stress, but *caused* by stress. Good grief!

I've seen too many people sitting at their desks and wearing their shoulders as earmuffs. Well, stay tuned folks: stiff necks, back and shoulder pain, and afternoon tension headaches to follow shortly!

And don't even get me going on shallow breathing! Well, okay, I have to at least mention it. The other problem with being under constant stress is that our breathing becomes shallower and shallower as the day progresses, depriving our organs, glands and muscles of oxygen—another vital requirement for healthy functioning.

Tomorrow at work, just for the heck of it, pay attention to your breathing and look in the mirror at where your shoulders rest before you start your day. Then stop at around 3:00 P.M. and check again. You may be surprised to find that you are taking shallow, little breaths from your rib cage instead of your diaphragm, and by 3:00 P.M., your shoulders are significantly higher. Shallow breathing causes your organs, glands and muscles, including those in your back, to become starved for oxygen. When stress causes you to hold tension in your lower back, or shoulders, *and* you're also breathing shallowly, you are restricting blood flow to your back and neck, and restricting the amount of oxygen getting through to your body parts. No wonder you are in chronic pain!

The bad news is that stress is unavoidable. The good news is that while you can't avoid stress, you *can* change your reaction to it, improving your health in the process. It takes a little planning and effort, but it's definitely possible.

Here are my two best techniques for stopping this vicious circle of nonstop stress dead in its tracks: 1) take conscious-breathing breaks and 2) laugh. They are so easy to use *and* you'll just love them!

Conscious-Breathing Breaks

Set your watch alarm or desktop calendar to go off once every hour. When the alarm goes off, *stop* what you're doing, sit tall in your chair, and close your eyes (so that you don't get distracted). Squeeze your shoulders up toward your ears and hold for a few seconds, then push them back as far as you can, arching your spine a little, and hold for a few seconds, and then let them rest in a normal position. Now inhale slowly, counting to five or six, and then exhale even more slowly, counting to seven or eight. Continue breathing slowly in this way for one to two minutes.

Everyone can devote at least a minute each hour to overall health. Why should you take these little breathing breaks?

1. This little conscious meditation on your breath will calm your mind and bring your breathing and heart rate back to normal.

2. Exhaling for longer than you inhale is a proven technique for lowering your blood pressure.

3. By sitting tall in your chair and stretching your shoulders a little, you restore circulation to your upper back and neck and improve your posture and ease of breathing as well.

4. These little conscious-breathing breaks circulate freshly oxygenated blood through your whole body, including your back, neck and shoulders, helping to restore proper functioning of organs, glands and muscles.

Now, wasn't that easy?

Clients have asked me if they need to keep up this pattern of hourly conscious-breathing breaks at home. Stopping to take a conscious-breathing break in the middle of driving your kids to soccer practice or while you're cooking dinner is not going to happen, so here is my recommendation: Once in the morning before you leave for work, and then once at night before you go to bed, stop and take a conscious-breathing break. Most people can fit these two breaks into their busy schedules, along with the hourly breaks at work. The powerful benefits you'll experience are worth the extra effort.

Even if you think you can't remember to take these breathing breaks, or can't fit your morning break in, leave yourself a note to complete your conscious-breathing break at night and make it a longer one, let's say five minutes' duration. This will definitely help you sleep better. And to help with your back pain, I recommend using the relaxation technique described in the next chapter for five minutes before you go to bed, while doing your evening conscious-breathing break. You'll sleep like a baby!

Laughter

Laughter is the best medicine. Truly, we all know that laughter makes us feel good. But aside from being fun, laughter has many health benefits, both mental and physical. A regular ten-minute laughter session can have a powerful impact on our overall health and well being. Laughter is gentle exercise for the lungs (which is really important for people who don't get regular aerobic exercise), and it enhances our core body workout. It also helps us fill our lungs and body with oxygen and clears breathing passages. Sustained laughter lowers your blood pressure, improves depression and mood, and boosts your immune system. [13-22]

Laughing makes you feel energized and refreshed because it releases endorphins. It also releases T-cells, the little Pac-Men of the body that eat up bad cells, such as any cancerous ones. Norman Cousins' account of using laughter to heal his own terminal disease has inspired millions of people. [23]

Researchers at California's Lorna Linda University announced the following findings at the 121st Annual Meeting of the American Physiological Society: "Laughing lowers levels of three stress hormones (dopac, cortisol, epinephrine) by 38, 39 and 70 percent respectively. Even anticipating laughter had the positive effect of boosting beta endorphins and human growth hormone, which has a positive effect on immunity."

So, stop those stress hormones from causing a car wreck in your body through comedy! When you feel yourself storing all that tension in your lower back, or if you feel the pressure building and those shoulders creeping up to your ears, take a laughing break! Read some funny jokes on the Internet or watch a funny movie or Comedy Central for a few minutes. Listen to an old Bill Cosby or Robin Williams recording while you're driving so you can avoid being stressed out by aggressive drivers. There are many ways to bring laughter back into your life, and I highly recommend making the effort. Not only will your back, neck and shoulders thank you, but your entire body will be happier!

Laughter also helps us relax, and relaxation is a major factor in relieving and preventing muscle pain. I've discovered many wonderful ways to relax muscles quickly, easing your back pain.

Chapter Seven

Why Muscle Relaxation Is the Key to Relief

"Those who say it cannot be done should not interrupt the person doing it."

—Chinese proverb

Muscle relaxation is my favorite topic. I could talk for hours on how important it is to relax all of the muscles in your back, but it's much more effective to show you. My "Three-Step Approach to Back, Neck and Sciatic Nerve Pain Relief" starts with this relaxation technique. Once your muscles are relaxed, you'll feel better, have less pain and be able to start steps two and three: stretching and strengthening.

In the following pages you will see a photo of me in my living room, in the position that works miracles for relaxing your back muscles. You will also find photos of my friend, Ned, who uses a pillow as a prop for this position so that he gets the same benefits and uses the proper posture.

To begin, sit on the floor next to your couch or a chair. Then, lie down onto your back, placing your buttocks right against the couch or chair so that your thighs are perpendicular to the floor and your lower legs are resting comfortably on the furniture. It looks like a sitting position, but you're on the floor in a sort of sideways sitting position. Now breathe… Continue breathing deeply for about five minutes.

In this position, your back is in a completely neutral position. The natural curve in your lower spine is intact and can rest, and all of the muscles in your back join in for some much needed R&R. Ahhhh… a lovely vacation for your back.

It's essential to make sure that your lower legs are completely resting on the couch or chair. If they are at all tense, this position will not work as well as it should. Also, the deep breathing brings freshly oxygenated blood to all of the muscles that are finally relaxing enough to *receive* some of the much-needed oxygen. I recommend counting slowly to 5 or 6 while inhaling and then, even more slowly, counting to 7 or 8 on your exhale.

This is the remedy that I mentioned earlier that I am passionate about sharing with the whole world! Once you try it, you'll also see the powerful effect of this one simple technique!

Now, if you can't lie flat on your back without arching your neck, place a small pillow or a rolled-up hand towel under your head, as Ned has done in the photographs. The reason this technique works so well is that your *entire* spine is in its natural, neutral position—and that includes your neck. Have someone check your posture to make sure you are in a comfortable, neutral position, using a pillow or towel if necessary, and then you'll be good to go.

Depending on your posture, you may need a bigger pillow. For instance, when my brother, Pat, was undergoing cancer treatments, he was stuck in a hunched over position in a chair for months, so he became very round shouldered. His back hurt all the time, so in addition to my niece and I using healing touch and Reiki on his back, I showed him this technique for relaxing his back muscles. At first, he needed a large pillow to achieve the correct position, but as his posture improved, he was able to use a smaller pillow. Pat also wore a back brace during the day—one like you see delivery men wear for lifting heavy packages. These two accommodations helped him to correct his posture and relieve his back pain so that he could begin an exercise program and gain back his strength. He's almost back to his old self again!

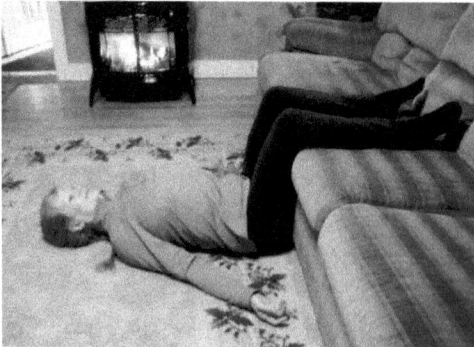

This is me with my back in a good position.

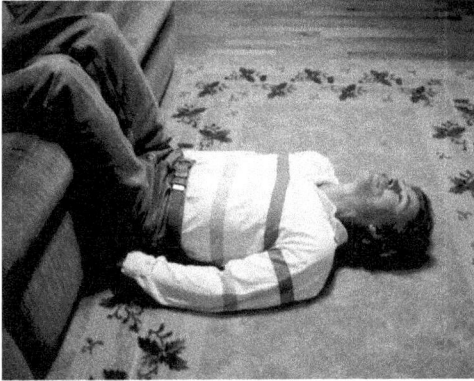

This is Ned with his neck arched—not good.

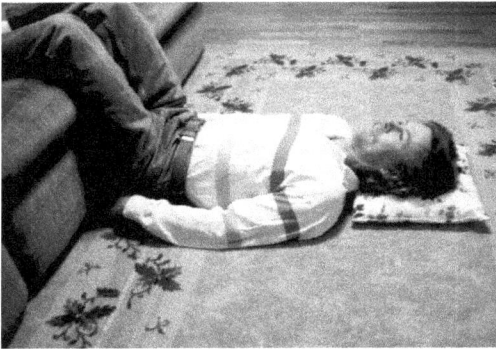

Here he is with a small pillow under his head—not his neck, his head. See what a big difference it makes?

I should say a word about gadgets for relaxing your back. The SacroWedgy® is a gadget based upon the principle of relaxing your muscles to find relief, as is the Back2Life®

massager (as seen on TV). I do not recommend spending the money for these expensive gadgets when you can find relief using your own couch and a blanket, *but* if you are one of those people who simply *must* have gadgets, I guess you could give them a try!

There are a couple of important reasons that my "Three-Step Approach to Relieving Back, Neck or Sciatic Nerve Pain" begins with relaxing all the muscles in your back. First, when back muscles are relaxed, this releases some of the pressure on all of your spinal nerves, which helps to ease the pain. We are often our own worst enemy. Our muscles automatically tense when we're in pain as a way to protect the area. However, this automatic response can cause even more pressure on the sciatic or other spinal nerves—making the pain worse! And the longer those muscles are tensed, the more difficult it becomes to relax them, causing a vicious circle of pain and more pain. Second, with less pain, you are able to stretch, massage and exercise to strengthen your back. Let's face it—no one wants to exercise when in excruciating pain!

Now that you know the number one best way in the universe to relax all of your back muscles to relieve your pain, you're ready for the second and third steps in my Three-Step Approach: stretching and strengthening!

Chapter Eight

The Top Seven Stretching Exercises for Back, Neck or Sciatic Nerve Pain Relief

"Whether you think you can or think you can't, you're right."

—Henry Ford

Here are photos and descriptions of the top six exercises I recommend for lasting relief of your back or neck pain, along with a neck-and-shoulder stretching exercise that can help alleviate neck pain and tension. I recommend that you pick two of them and make them a part of your daily routine. As I mentioned earlier, the best way to keep your pain from becoming a frequent visitor is to learn the tools of my Three-Step Approach and then integrate them into your life. If you know how to relax those muscles, the best stretches to help keep them flexible and healthy, and the best way to strengthen your back, then you have the tools to relieve your pain. It's up to you to make using them a part of your life and prevent the pain from coming back.

I know that some of you won't take these words to heart. It's happened before, when I've given these tools to a client and he faithfully completes all the stretches and exercises for a while, but then starts to feel great and thinks it's okay to skip a day or two, then a week or a month. The next thing you know, I'm getting a call because he is in pain again and needs help. I can't emphasize enough how important it is to do the exercises regularly.

Stretching Exercise 1: Through the Hole

The first stretching exercise is called "Through the Hole" because you thread your arm through the hole between your legs like a thread being pushed through a needle. Don't worry if you can't do this stretch without pain; I have included a modified version so that you can get some relief without more pain!

This easy-to-do exercise stretches all of the muscles around your hip, lower back and buttocks. When you are in a lot of pain, do your five minutes of muscle relaxation then follow with this exercise.

Lie on your back on the floor with knees bent and your feet flat, about hip distance apart.

Cross your right ankle over your left thigh, and bring your left leg up off the floor, straightening it and pointing the toe if you can (it's okay to have your left knee bent if that's more comfortable for you).

Now reach through the hole between your legs with your right arm and reach around the back of your left leg with your left arm until your hands can clasp and gently pull your legs closer to your body.

Check to make sure that your head is still on the floor and your neck is not arched. Tuck your chin in toward your chest a little to straighten out your neck, or place a small pillow under your head as in the photo below.

Breathe deeply for one to two minutes while gently stretching.

Now lower your left leg and repeat with the opposite leg.

Note: Make sure that your ankle is not resting on your knee. Place it on your thigh (as in the picture) or on your shin, but keep it off the knee.

Remember to stretch *gently*. Only pull your leg as far as you can without pain. A little discomfort is okay, but not pain.

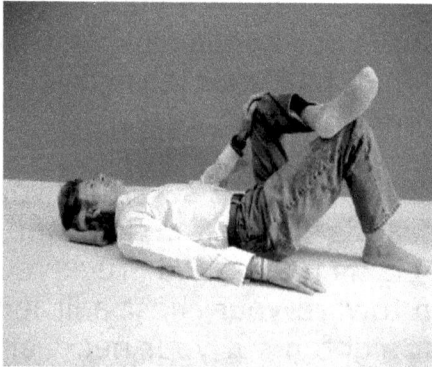

This is a modified position with foot on the floor. Gently press your left knee away from you.

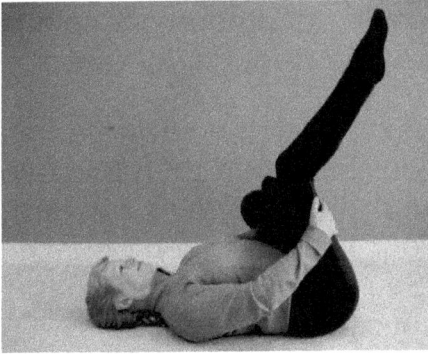

Full stretch

Stretching Exercise 2: Downward Facing Dog Yoga Pose

Practicing yoga has many health benefits, especially for stretching and strengthening your neck, legs and back. The downward facing dog pose balances the entire bladder meridian, which, according to Eastern medicine, controls the back, neck, buttocks, back of the legs and outside edges of the feet. In Western terms, it stretches the hamstring, spine and shoulder muscles. Most people love doing the Downward Facing Dog because it feels really, really good.

Begin by standing tall with your feet hip distance apart. As you inhale, lengthen your spine all the way up through your neck.

Next, stretch your arms up above your head and then fold over from your hips, reaching forward. Keep your back flat; don't hunch it! (See photo.). It helps if you stick your butt out a little.

When you've folded forward as far as you can with a flat back, let your head and arms relax.

Rest in this forward bend for one deep breath to encourage your spine to relax completely.

Now bend your knees so that you can bring your palms to the floor on either side of your feet.

Walk your hands out on your mat until you look like an inverted V, raising your hips toward the ceiling while stretching heels toward the floor at the same time.

Breathe deeply for one to two minutes, relaxing further with each breath.

Bend your knees slightly and reverse the exercise, coming back to a standing position by slowly rolling up one vertebra at a time

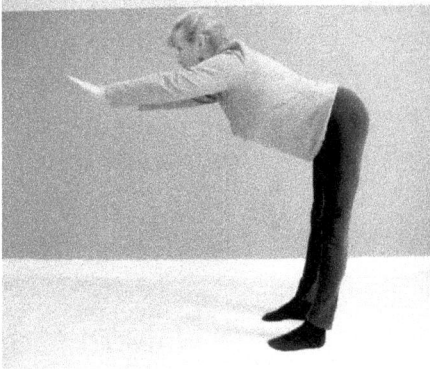

Folding down into position with a *flat back*

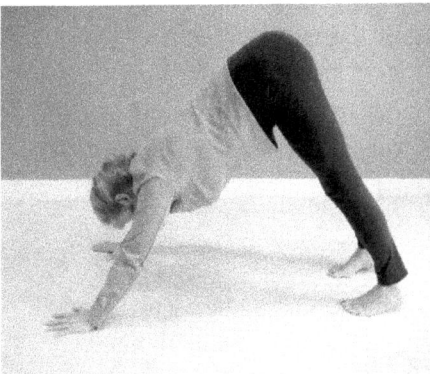

Downward Facing Dog Pose

Stretching Exercise 3: Sleeping Pigeon

Sleeping Pigeon is one of my favorites. This yoga pose stretches all of the muscles along the path that your sciatic nerve travels. I find this particular yoga pose elicits the largest number of OMG! responses—after people have done the relaxation technique in the previous chapter, of course.

Begin in the Downward Facing Dog pose with your weight on all four limbs, stretching your buttocks up toward the ceiling while at the same time stretching your heels toward the floor. If this is not possible for you, begin kneeling in a sort of table position, with your back flat (see photo.)

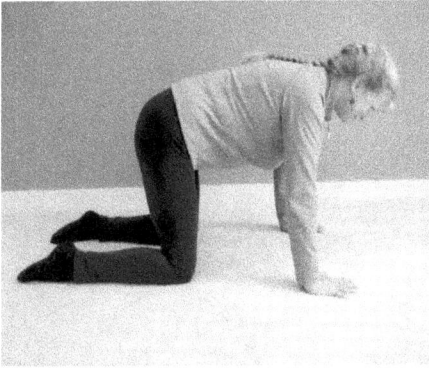

Modified start from table position

Bring your right knee forward and place it between your hands on the floor with the lower leg angled slightly toward your left wrist. Lower your body down on top of the legs as far as possible (you can hold yourself up with your hands or arms) and stretch the left leg out straight behind you.

Relax and breathe deeply for two minutes.

To come out of the position, place your palms under your shoulders, inhale, and press into your palms as you lift your body back to Downward Facing Dog Pose or back to table position.

Repeat with the opposite leg.

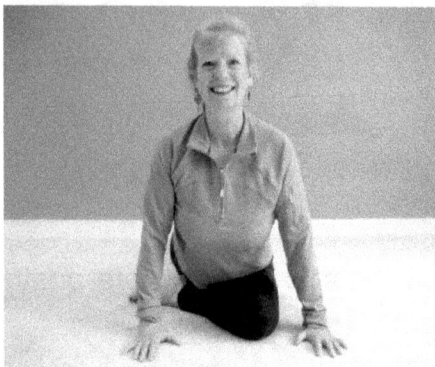

Sleeping Pigeon modified

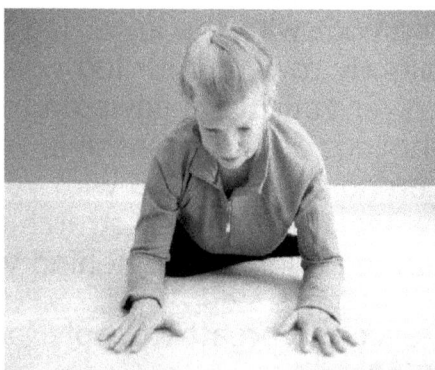

Modification 2

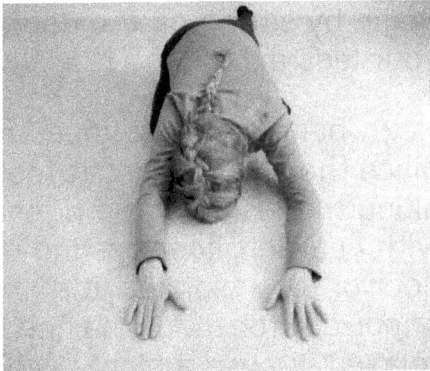

Sleeping Pigeon full stretch

Stretching Exercise 4: Head-to-Knee Stretch Using Acupressure Points B 53 and 54

In the hollow behind your knee are the 53rd and 54th acupressure points located along the bladder meridian ("B" before the number is for bladder). Applying pressure to these points can help relieve pain in the back and the backs of the legs, leg numbness or coldness, spasms, rheumatism, stiffness in the back and neck and arthritis in the knee. This head-to-knee exercise stretches the lumbar sacral area of the spine as well as the hamstring (East meets West again).

Begin by sitting on the floor with your legs extended.

Next, bend your left knee and place the sole of the left foot along the inside of the right thigh with your left knee resting on the floor or on a blanket. It's important for that left knee to be relaxed, so use a blanket or pillow under it if needed.

Inhale and lift your arms, stretching them upward. Then turn your torso to the right and face your right leg.

While exhaling, stretch forward over your leg *with a flat back* as far as you can and then relax your arms and head.

Place your left fist in the hollow behind the right knee, placing pressure on the points, or, if your knee doesn't go all the way down when you're in this stretch, you can press your fingers into the hollow behind your knee.

Breathe into the stretch for 1 to 2 minutes, deepening the stretch as you breathe.

To come back up to sitting tall, bring your back into a flat position again, then inhale and lift your torso, neck and head up. Release your fist, and extend your left leg.

Repeat on the other side.

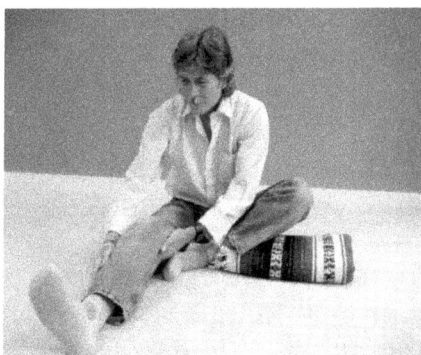

Resting your knee on a blanket and pressing fingers into B 53 & 54.

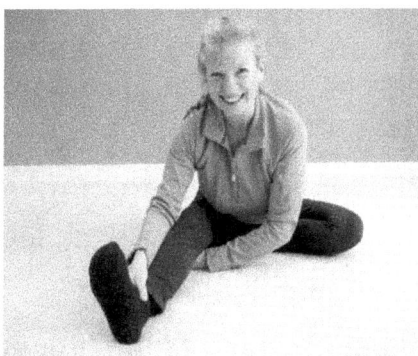

Flat back, stretching out over leg and smiling ☺

Stretching Exercise 5: Sitting Pigeon

Sitting Pigeon is a way to get almost the same stretch as Sleeping Pigeon, but it can be done while sitting in a chair or any time that you can't or don't want to get down on the floor. It can be done easily while sitting in a meeting or working at your desk.

First, sit tall in your chair and relax your shoulders.

Then rest your right ankle over your left thigh. Make sure you don't have the ankle resting on your knee.

Now, take hold of the seat of your chair with both hands and lean forward with a flat back. You'll feel the stretch in your right hip, thigh and buttocks.

Breathe deeply for one to two minutes and then switch legs.

This is especially recommended for times when you have to sit in long meetings. It will help keep those muscles stretched so that they don't tense up on you. Repeat every hour if you can.

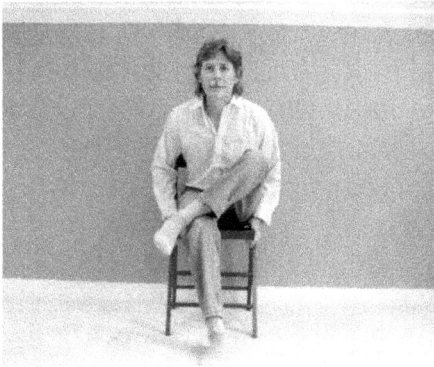

Note: I have mentioned several times in the above exercises the importance of keeping your back flat and I'd like to explain here why that's so important. If you have osteoporosis or disks that are damaged, bending forward without a flat back, or rounding your back in some of these stretches, can cause the front inside portion of your disk to crumble a little more and that's definitely not something that you want to do! So, to be on the safe side, whether you have osteoporosis or not, it's just good practice to always use a flat back when doing a forward bend.

Stretching Exercise 6: Piriformis Syndrome Stretch

Here's a great one for those of you who have piriformis syndrome. (Note, too, that the Sitting Pigeon is a great fix for your piriformis syndrome pain.) This exercise is an amazing little technique that helps release all of the tension in your piriformis muscle through a simple self-massage.

Lie on your back with knees bent and feet flat on floor.

Place your fists or back of your hands under the center of each buttock.

Now, inhale as you roll your knees gently to the right, then exhale slowly while using your abdominal muscles to pull your knees back to the center.

On your next breath, roll your knees to the other side.

Breathe deeply and continue slowly rolling your knees from one side to the other for 1 to 2 minutes. Be sure to keep your feet flat and knees bent throughout this entire exercise.

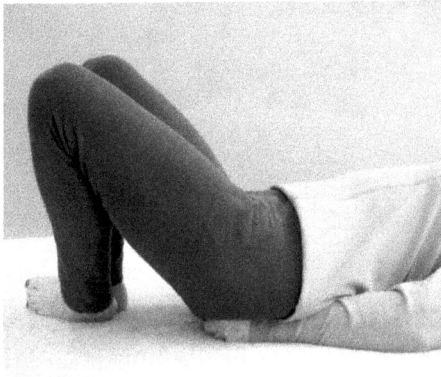

Dropping knees to the left with the fists placed under buttocks

You can also use my **Tension Tamer Balls** (*http://bit.ly/notension*) for this self-massage. You can place these handy devices under your buttocks instead of using your hands, making it a little easier to relax your arms and shoulders. Some people use tennis balls, but I find them too firm—they hurt!

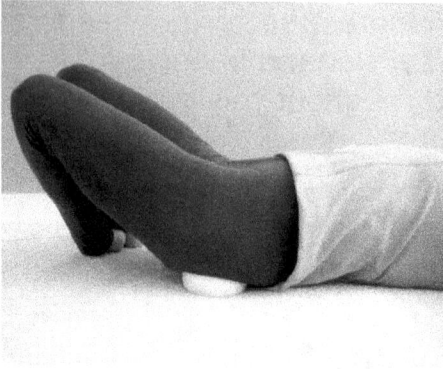

Stretching Exercise 7: Neck-and-Shoulder Stretch

Neck and shoulder relief is at your fingertips! This is my top technique for keeping neck and shoulder tension at bay. You can do this exercise at work, travelling, or anywhere that you feel the need. This simple exercise relaxes your shoulder and neck muscles while at the same time pressing on vital acupressure points that help to relieve neck pain and headaches.

Begin by sitting tall in your chair. Lengthen your spine all the way up through your neck.
Now reach your hands around to the thick muscle at the back of

your neck where it meets your shoulders. You can feel this muscle on each side as it's very thick. Curl your fingers around it and squeeze as hard as you can manage without pain. Remember some discomfort is okay, but not pain.

Inhale deeply, counting to 5 or 6, then exhale longer, counting to 6 or 7 as you continue to squeeze for 1 to 2 minutes.

Now, slowly release the pressure on that muscle and give it a little massage. You'll notice that it's warmer now because all of the blood is flowing nicely. When muscles are tensed, the circulation is restricted, but this exercise relaxes the neck and shoulder muscles and promotes good circulation to the area (that's why it starts to feel warmer).

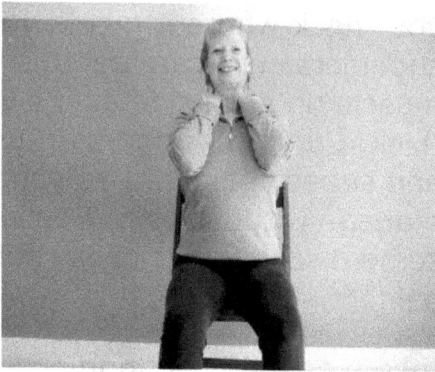

The Neck-and-Shoulder Stretch is such a great preventative that I recommend repeating it every hour if you're one of the many people who carry their stress around in that "stress backpack."

If you find it difficult to do it on both sides at the same time, you can squeeze one side at a time for at least a minute before switching sides.

If you tend to get afternoon neck pain and tension headaches, do this exercise. Then simply move your hands an inch or two up the sides of your neck and squeeze the thick muscle there while breathing deeply.

Chapter Nine

Seven Exercises to Strengthen Your Core Body—All of the Muscles Surrounding Your Back and Neck

"A bear, however hard he tries, grows tubby without exercise."

—A.A. Milne, "Teddy Bear"

The stronger the muscles surrounding your back and neck are, the more support you have as you stand, sit, and move your body. These core muscles can be strengthened using the seven exercises presented here.

Exercise 1: The Cat/Cow Stretch

The Cat/Cow Stretch is one of my all-time favorites. This is a basic, simple exercise where you completely flex and extend your spine. I recommend completing the Cat/Cow Stretch every morning when you get out of bed so that you start your day off on a good note.

Often, our backs are a little stiff from lying in bed all night, and then if we twist slightly while reaching into our closet, or move a little too fast while putting on our jacket, we feel that unforgettable twinge...

Well, warming up your spine a little before you do anything else will help solve that problem. (The Cat/Cow Stretch is also a perfect warm-up before doing any back strengthening exercises.)

Get on the floor and position yourself on all fours, with your hands lined up with your shoulders and your knees lined up with your hips so that you look like a table. Inhale deeply.

As you exhale, start the movement by tucking your tailbone under, lifting and rounding your back, and bringing your chin toward your chest. You will look like a cat stretching.

On your inhale, tilt your tailbone up, releasing the abdomen down toward the floor and bringing your chest forward, raising your head slightly. You will resemble a cow with your belly hanging down.

Repeat for five or six deep, full breaths.

Remember to always start the movement with your tailbone to prevent straining your neck.

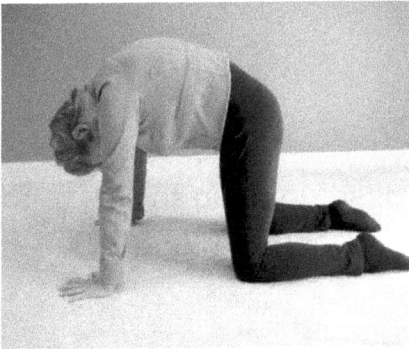

Cat stretch

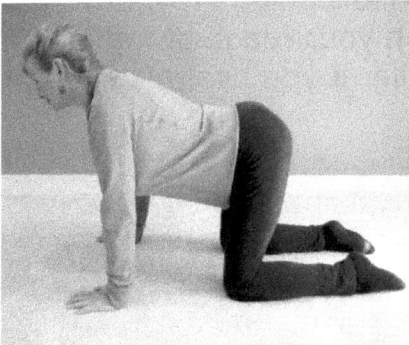

Cow stretch

If you have pain in your wrists, you can do this exercise with rolled up hand towels placed underneath your palms. Relax your fingers and curl them toward the floor.

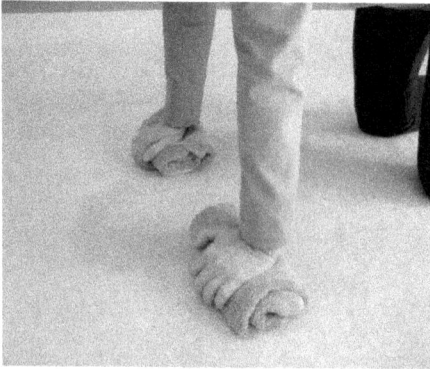

Using rolled up hand towels to take the pressure off your wrists.

The Cat/Cow Stretch can also be done while leaning on your forearms, although your range of movement will be smaller if you use this variation.

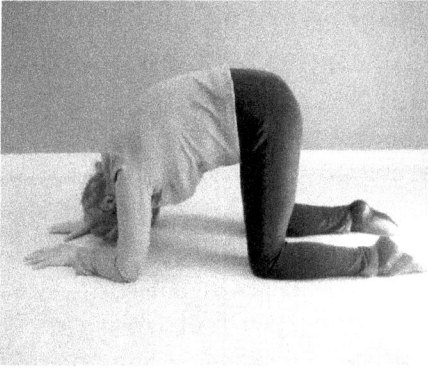

Exercise 2: The Bridge

The Bridge Exercise, used by physical therapists, chiropractors, osteopaths and yoga teachers everywhere, is the best lower-back strengthening exercise there is.

Begin lying on your back on the floor with your feet flat and knees bent. Your feet should be hip distance apart.

As you inhale, tuck in your tailbone, and then lift one vertebra at a time as you slowly raise into the position pictured below. When you are in a good strong bridge position, your feet will be pressing into the floor, and your thighs, abs and buttock muscles will be nice and tight.

Breathe deeply in this position for at least thirty seconds, then come back down slowly on an exhale, one vertebra at a time. Rest, and go back up into the bridge position again for another 30 seconds.

Work up to remaining in this position for the entire minute, but that may take a while so go as slowly as you need to. You can begin with doing it for just five seconds if that's where you need to start.

Remember, in any exercise program, it's important to listen to your body. If it hurts, or you feel you should stop what you're doing and rest, please do so.

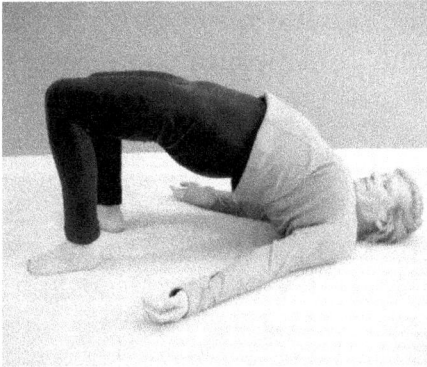

Full Bridge Pose

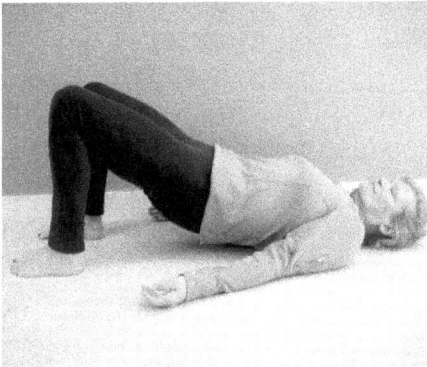

Saggy Bridge—try not to sag...

Exercise 3: The Single-Leg Stretch

The Pilates exercise called the Single-Leg Stretch strengthens your lower back muscles *and* your abdominal muscles, helping to build core muscles, stamina and support for your back.

Begin lying on your back with your feet flat on the floor and your knees bent.

Next, bend your right knee and bring it toward your chest so that you can place your hands around it and fully extend your left leg, raising it slightly off the floor.

Next, raise your head and shoulders by using your abdominal muscles.

Now, inhale in two short puffs as you use your hands to pull your bent knee toward your chin twice. Exhale, blowing all the air out of your lungs as you switch legs to perform the exercise again on the other side. Repeat the exercise six times in each direction, and remember to pull your knee toward your chest and not out toward your shoulders.

Next, lower your head, and hug your knees into your chest while rocking a little and breathing deeply.

Note: This exercise can be done without lifting your upper body off the floor at first until you build a little strength in your core. It's important not to strain your neck while trying to build up your strength!

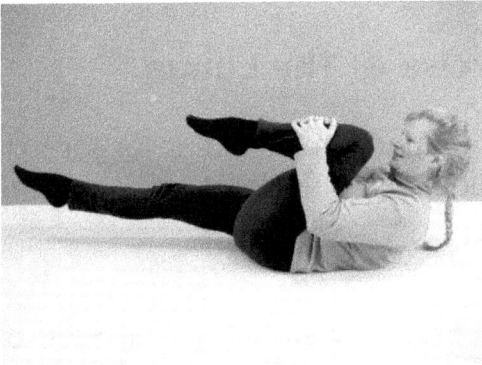

Here I am smiling again!

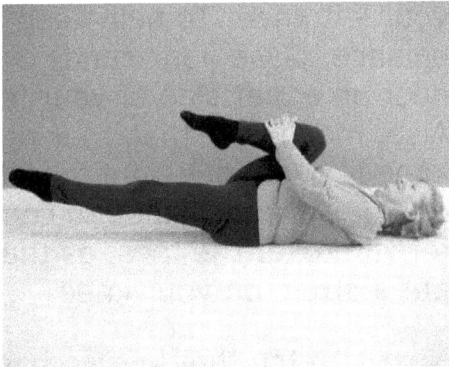

Modified position with head resting on floor

Now we should talk a little about the iliopsoas muscle. This muscle is on the front of your hip and it's a difficult one to stretch and strengthen. However, it's also one that can cause some pretty severe sciatic nerve pain, so it's important to stretch it.

Exercise 4: The Lunge

The Lunge is excellent for stretching the iliopsoas muscle.

Begin by standing tall. Step back with your left leg—as far back as you can—and drop down onto your left knee. To help keep your balance, place your hands on the floor on either side of your feet. Also, make sure that your right knee is over your right foot. You do not want that knee to come forward over the toes, as that will put a strain on your knee.

Next, stretch that left leg back a little bit more. You can keep your hands on the floor if you are comfortable there, or bring them up onto your right thigh.

Inhale as you stretch your pelvic area downward toward the floor. You should feel this stretch in your left groin and hip.

Breathe deeply in this position, stretching farther—as far as you can without causing pain.

Continue stretching for about a minute. Then repeat the exercise on the other side.

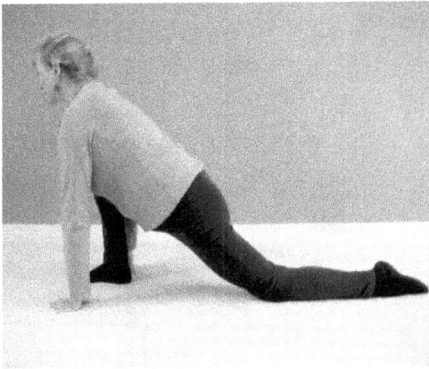

Notice how my core is lowered toward the floor.

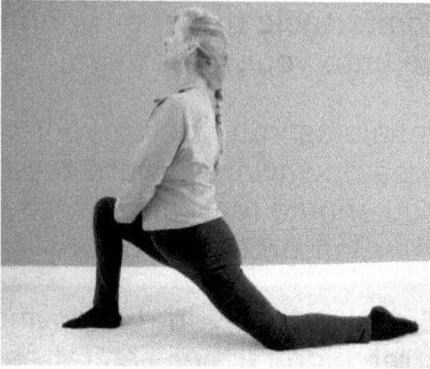

Hands on thighs

Exercise 5: The Crunch

"Crunch" is not necessarily a bad word. There are tiny crunches you can do to strengthen your core body without straining any muscles. Too many military style crunches can strain your iliopsoas muscle, however, so that's why we're going to do a slightly different version.

Begin lying on your back on the floor with your knees bent and feet flat about hip distance apart.

Inhale deeply and then exhale as you squeeze your abdominal

muscles to raise your upper body *slightly* off the floor. Hold this position for two seconds.

Lower yourself back down to the floor slowly. Repeat.

Note: You can either place your hands on your belly or your chest during this exercise.

Start with anywhere from two to four crunches. Then, as you become stronger, you can build up to six reps. Remember to go slowly and make your abs do all of the work. Keep checking that you have no tension in your neck during this exercise.

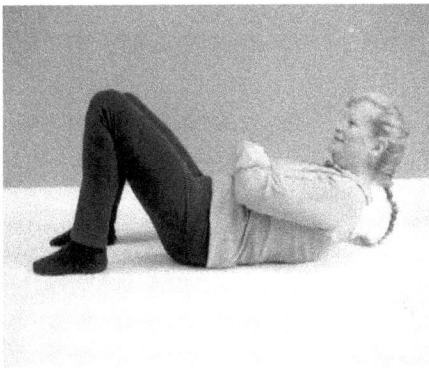

Let your abs do all the work!

Exercise 6: Pilates "Swimming"

Swimming is an excellent exercise for strengthening your whole body, and the **Pilates swimming** exercise gives you its benefits without your having to get wet. This exercise is a great one for strengthening your upper and lower back while loosening your hip and shoulder joints.

Begin by lying on the floor, face down, with your arms extended above your head about shoulder width apart. Your legs should be extended about hip distance apart. Keep your chin on the mat as you look forward.

Inhale as you lift and stretch your right arm and your left leg at the same time. Exhale and lower them.

Then inhale and lift your left arm and right leg. Exhale and lower them.

Repeat five or six times.

Note: As you do this exercise, keep your arms, legs, and spine straight. You're doing a stretch, not a leg lift. Also, do not turn your head from side to side because that puts a strain on your neck. If you feel any tension in your lower back, please tighten your buttocks to remove the tension.

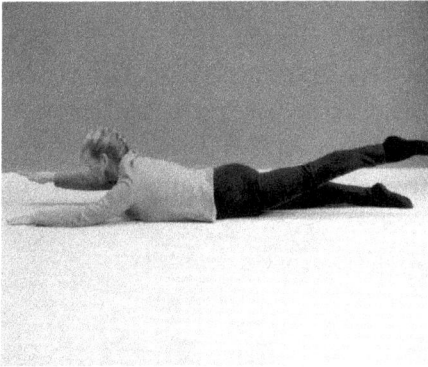

Swim away from the sharks...

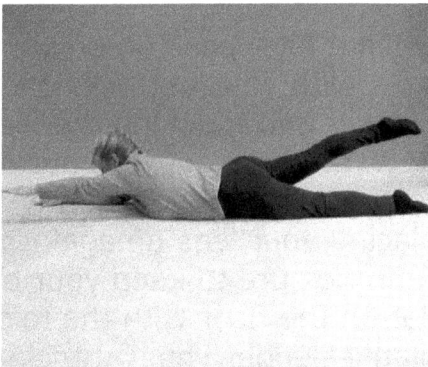

and into better health!

Exercise 7: Shoulder Stand

A great exercise for strengthening your shoulders and neck is the yoga inversion called **shoulder stand**. Now I know some of you are shuddering at the thought of completing an inversion, which will require you to be upside down, but hear me out. I'm not going to ask you to do anything that you can't do. Haven't I given you modifications for all of the exercises so far to make sure that everyone can do them? This one starts out quite easy and I think you'll find that you really like it when you give it a try.

Start out by placing a folded blanket next to a solid wall.

Lie in a fetal position on your right side, with your buttocks on the blanket and touching the wall. Now, stretch your legs out as you roll on to your back, gently placing your legs up against the wall. Be sure to keep your back flat on the floor with the folded blanket under your buttocks. Your butt should be pressing right up to the wall. If it's not, then just schooch (very scientific term) yourself up against the wall.

Keep your arms alongside your body with the palms facing upward. Remain here, breathing deeply for about three minutes.

As you start to feel more comfortable in this modified yoga shoulder stand, you can add more blankets to your pile so that your butt is lifted higher and you feel more weight on your shoulders.

When you're ready, you can even bend your knees and place your feet flat against the wall, pressing into your feet to raise up onto your shoulders a little more. You can take one foot away from the wall for a few seconds, then put it back into position and remove the other.

Only when you feel very strong are you ready for the full shoulder stand pose away from the wall. I have added a photo of this pose; however, it's an advanced pose and should not be attempted without personal instruction from a yoga teacher.

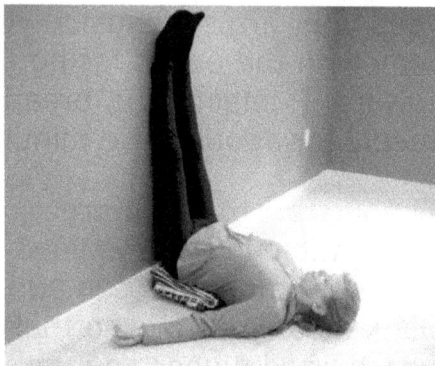

Legs up the wall—easy inversion

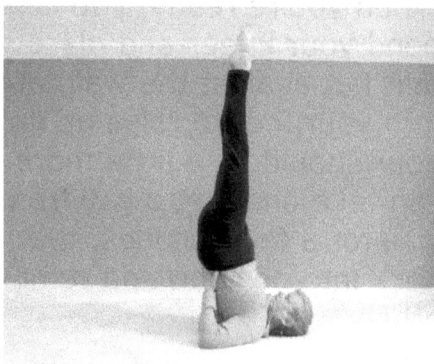

Photo of full shoulder stand. (Make sure you tuck your shirt in first :O)

Bonus Exercise: The Forearm Plank

Here is a bonus, advanced exercise for those who are looking for a bit more of a challenge. The **Forearm Plank** strengthens your entire core, providing more stabilization for your back.

Begin by lying face down on the floor. Bring your elbows under your shoulders while keeping your forearms and hands flat on the floor, about shoulder width apart. It's important to position your forearms parallel to your body.

Next, curl your toes and lift your body into a plank position—only instead of having your weight on your hands, as in a traditional yoga plank position, you are balancing on your forearms. This makes the pose a little more challenging while also making it possible for anyone with weak wrists to do the exercise.

Hold this position for several seconds, then rest for a breath or two, and repeat. Work up to holding the pose for at least ten seconds, repeating the position twice.

Note: Make sure that your lower back is not swayed but flat. If your back tends to drop toward the floor, simply raise your hips slightly toward the ceiling to protect your lower back.

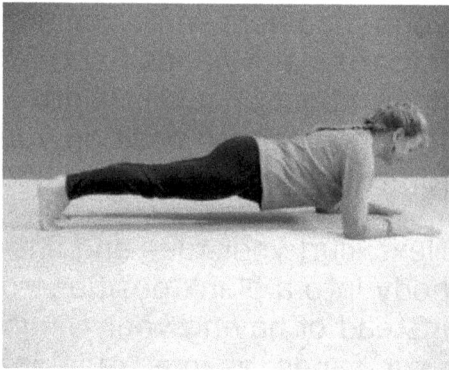

Chapter Ten

Easy Lifestyle Changes for Today and the Rest of Your Life

"The road to success is always under construction."

—Lily Tomlin

I know that both Oprah and my sister will be very unhappy with this recommendation, but **high heels** *are not good for our backs, so you should avoid wearing them.* There, I said it. Lightning did not strike me down nor did the roof cave in.

For proper posture and alignment, wear heels no higher than one inch. I'm happy with this recommendation because I've always been very uncomfortable in three- or four-inch heels; however, I know many women who feel naked without their high heels. The problem is that high heels not only throw off our posture and alignment, but can cause foot injuries, which then aggravate back pain. Today, all the doctors I know recommend pumps or a similar shoe with a small heel to avoid these problems.

Sitting for long periods of time can aggravate back pain, too. Truck drivers, computer workers and others who must sit for long periods have more back issues than manual laborers do!

If you work at a desk all day, make sure you can sit tall in your chair without slouching. Keep your workstation set up to provide good posture and ease of movement while working. When I work at a desk, I find that resting my feet on a small box helps me sit more comfortably. The only problem is that when I first started doing this, I had to stop the cleaners from tossing it into the trash each night! Eventually, I made a large sign that said "DO NOT REMOVE" and placed the box on my chair when I left each day.

Get up and walk around as often as you can. If you have a headset for your telephone, then you can pace around the desk every time you're on the phone. Take the long way to the bathroom and copier so that you get a few extra steps in. Anything that you can do to add movement and stretching will be of benefit in reducing your pain and tension.

The key is to take regular movement breaks to stretch. Of course, truck drivers must stop to use the bathroom facilities every couple of hours, and people who work at computers need to get out of their chairs occasionally as well. However, there are two simple stretches, a variation of the Cat/Cow Stretch and a Seated Hamstring Stretch, that can be done while seated in your chair.

Chair Exercise 1: The Seated Cat/Cow Stretch

The Seated Cat/Cow Stretch helps to release tension in the muscles along your spinal nerves. It takes only a minute or two to do, yet can save hours of pain, so "just do it!"

Remember to keep your bent knee above your ankle, not over your toes. And don't forget to breathe!

Sit tall in your chair with your feet flat on the floor.

Inhale deeply and arch your back, tilting your chin up slightly.

Exhale slowly as you begin to curl your spine starting at the tailbone, hunching forward slightly.

Be sure to breathe deeply and start the movement each time with your tailbone so that you don't strain your neck.

This Seated Cat/Cow Stretch warms up your spine and maintains flexibility when you have to sit for long periods.

Chair Exercise 2: Hamstring Stretch

The other exercise I recommend for people who sit most of the day is the Hamstring Chair Stretch. This stretch helps reduce the tension in your lower back and can be done any time you are seated.

Sit up straight, close to the edge of your chair. Keeping your left leg bent with the foot flat on the floor, and your left knee positioned over your foot, stretch your right leg out so that only your heel is on the floor. Then, "dig in your heel" by pressing it against the floor.

Next, hold onto the seat of your chair with both hands and bend over gently until you feel the muscles in the back of your leg stretching.

Breathe and stretch for about a minute, then switch legs.

Lifting heavy cartons or carrying heavy bags can also aggravate your sciatic nerve pain, so if you carry a heavy purse or briefcase, try to downsize, or use a backpack that is ergonomically designed. If you must lift heavy packages for your job, wear a lifting belt and make sure you bend your knees and lift from your legs without twisting. Twisting while lifting is the worst thing you can do for your back. It puts your disks into an unsupported position, risking injury.

And remember the importance of resting and relaxing your back muscles. Complete the relaxation exercise in Chapter Seven at least once or twice a day to give your muscles a chance to relax completely.

Many people don't realize that **the way you walk** makes a huge difference in whether or not you aggravate your back pain. I recommend walking like John Wayne—seriously! In the John Wayne walk, you begin each step by moving your hip bone forward. If you concentrate on starting each step with your hip and not your knee, while also squaring your shoulders and lifting your head, you'll be in proper alignment. Bet you didn't know that was why the old cowboy walked that way, did you? He was ahead of his time...

The John Wayne walk will make your hips sway a bit more, and it may feel awkward at first, but I recommend practicing at home. Walk slowly and gradually start to walk this way when you're outside. In time, the John Wayne walk will become second nature.

Being **overweight** puts a strain on your lower back. Even as little as ten pounds of excess weight can cause back or leg pain. It's important to eat nurturing food and get plenty of exercise to keep your weight down.

For all of you type A personalities who rush through your day from one task to another and who resist exercise because you think that you can't possibly fit one more thing into your busy schedules, think again! Multitasking is not dead. An exhilarating march in place while brushing your teeth, a tango while setting the table, lunges while waiting for your copies at the photocopying machine or while on line at the supermarket, are all examples of simple, yet powerful ways to "fit" fitness into your daily routines without taking time away from family or career.

And the best suggestion I can make for a healthy diet is to keep a food log.

Write down every food or beverage you put into your mouth for seven days. You will be shocked. Most of us underestimate how much we eat and drink and overestimate how much we exercise. Many of my clients have lost weight simply by keeping a food log because it made them aware of just how many calories they were consuming. When you see how much you are eating, you can easily begin to make simple changes, such as substituting an apple for the pile of cheese and crackers you eat while making dinner, or eliminating any mindless snacking during work hours. You can make these simple changes without feeling deprived. Try it!

So, Now What?

It is my sincere desire that everyone who is suffering with long-term back pain will use the information in this book to begin taking their health care into their own hands and find a natural method to relieve pain, strengthen their muscles and prevent that pain in the backside from ever coming back again!

There are so many options for relieving back pain that you surely can find one that resonates with you. I've given you at least a little bit of information on several techniques and approaches that my research has found work very well for healing back pain. Please don't be afraid to try several of the healing therapies covered in this book. After all, your Western doctor has tried several different medications, tests, exercises, etc., hasn't he? Yet, you still have your back pain. Why not give the same consideration to Eastern medical practices—those that have been working for centuries? What have you got to lose, except your back pain?!

After reading this book, you now know that you do not need to suffer with back pain. Take back your life today!

And if you'd like more training from me personally, here is a link to my *Ultimate Back Neck and Sciatic Nerve Pain Relief Coaching Program* (http://bit.ly/EndofPain). In this program, we'll work one-on-one via Skype or telephone to discover exactly what's causing your pain and how to resolve it once and for all.

Best of health—especially back health—to you all,

Kathi

Notes

1. Hart, L.G., R.A. Deyo, D.C. Cherkin. "Physician Office Visits for Low Back Pain: Frequency, Clinical Evaluation, and Treatment Patterns from a U.S. National Survey." *Spine* (1995); 20:11-9.

2. Deyo, R.A., S.K. Mirza, B.I. Martin. "Back Pain Prevalence and Visit Rates: Estimates from U.S. National Surveys, 2002." *Spine* (2006); 31:2724-7.

3. National Institutes of Health.

4. Carey, T.S., A.T. Evans, N. M. Hadler, G. Lieberman, W.D. Kalsbeek, A.M. Jackman, et al. "Acute Severe Low Back Pain: A Population-Based Study of Prevalence and Care-Seeking." *Spine* (1996); 21:339-44.

5. Vallfors, B. "Acute, Subacute and Chronic Low Back Pain: Clinical Symptoms, Absenteeism and Working Environment." *Scandinavian Journal of Rehabilitation Medical Supplement* (1985); 11:1-98.

6. Andersson, GB. "Epidemiological Features of Chronic Low-Back Pain." *Lancet* (1999); 354:581-5.

7. This total represents only the more readily identifiable costs for medical care, workers compensation payments and time lost from work. It does not include costs associated with lost personal income due to acquired physical limitation resulting from a back problem and lost employer productivity due to employee medical absence. In Project Briefs: Back Pain Patient Outcomes Assessment Team (BOAT). In MEDTEP Update, Vol. 1 Issue 1, Agency for Health Care Policy and Research, Rockville, MD, Summer 1994.

8. http://search.barnesandnoble.com/EFT-for-PTSD/Gary-Craig/e/9781604150407

9. "Superficial Heat and Cold: How to Maximise the Benefits." *The Physician and Sportsmedicine* (1994); vol. 22(12):65-74.

10. Dana Farber. "Inside The Institute." *QiGong* (Sept. 14, 2004); Volume 9, Issue 19.

11. Jahnke, Roger, OMOD, Linda Larkey, PhD; Carol Rogers, APRN-BC, CNOR, PhD; Jennifer Etnier, PhD; Fang Lin, MS. "The Science of Health Promotion: A Comprehensive Review of Health Benefits of Qigong and Tai Chi." *Health Promotion Journal* (July/August 2010); Vol. 24, No. 6.

12. University of Alberta (2007, May 18). "Chronic Pain Can Impair Memory." *ScienceDaily.* Retrieved November 2, 2010, from http://www.sciencedaily.com releases/2007/05/070517142536.htm Some information was also found on www.MayoClinic.com

13. Berk, I. S., S. A. Tan, W.F. Fry, B.J. Napier, J.W. Lee, R.W. Hubbard, J.E. Lewis, and W.C. Eby. "Neuroendocrine and Stress Hormone Changes During Mirthful Laughter." *The American Journal of the Medical Sciences* (1989); 298:390-396.

14. Berk, I. S., S. A. Tan, S.L. Nehlsen-Cannarella, B.J. Napier, J.W. Lee, R.W. Hubbard, J.E. Lewis, W.C. Eby, W.F. Fry. "Humor Associated Laughter Decreases Cortisol and Increases Spontaneous Lymphocyte

Blastogenesis." *Clinical Research* (1988); 36:435A.

15. Berk, L.S., S.A. Tan, B.J. Napier, W.C. Eby. "Stress of Mirthful Laughter Modifies Natural Killer Cell Activity." *Clinical Research* (1989); 37:115A.

16. Besedovsky, H.O., A.E. Rey, A.E., and E. Sorkin. "Immune-neuroendocrine Interactions." *The Journal of Immunology* (1985); 135(2):750s-754s.

17. Bioten, F.A. "The effects of Emotional Behavior on Components of the Respiratory Cycle." *Biological Psychology* (1998); 49 (1-2): 29-.

18. Dillon, K., B. Minchoff, K. Baker. "Positive Emotional States and the Enhancement of the Immune System." *International Journal of Psychiatry in Medicine* (1985); 15:13-18.

19. J. R. Dunn interview with P. Derks. "Humor Health Letter (1992); 4:1-7. *Psychology* (1998) 49 (1-2):29-51.

20. W. F. Fry, C. Rader. "The Respiratory Components of Mirthful Laughter." *Journal of Biological Psychology* (1977) 19:39-50.

21. Fry, William F., Jr. "The Physiologic Effects of Humor, Mirth, and Laughter." *Journal of the American Medical Association* (1992); 267(13):1857.

22. Kamei, T., H. Kumano, S. Masumura. "Changes of Immunoregulatory Cells Associated with Psychological Stress and Humor." *Perceptual and Motor Skills* (1997); 84 (3 pt. 2): 1296-8.

23. Cousins, Norman. *Head First: The Biology of Hope.* New York: Dutton, 1989.

Recommended Resources

Tom Papke, PT
   http://capitalmetrophysicaltherapy.com/

Dr. Philip Grover
   http://www.facebook.com/people/Philip-Grover/1638496701

Audrey Herrick
   http://awakenhealingarts.com

Borysenko, Joan, PhD, and Miroslav Borysenko, MD. *The Power of the Mind to Heal: Renewing Body, Mind and Spirit.* Carlsbad, CA: Hay House, 2004.

Chopra, Deepak, MD. *Perfect Health: The Complete Mind/Body Guide.*
Dean, Carolyn. *Future Health Now Encyclopedia.*

Hanna, Thomas. *Somatics: Reawakening the Mind's Control of Movement, Flexibility, and Health.* Cambridge, MA: Da Capo Books, 2004.

Hay, Louise. *You Can Heal Your Life.* Carlsbad, CA: Hay House, 1994.

Hyman, Mark. *The UltraMind Solution.* New York: Harmony Books, 1990.

Sarno, John, MD. *The MindBody Prescription: Healing the Body, Healing the Pain.* New York: Warner Books, 1999.

Weismann, Darren, DC. *The Power of Infinite Love and Gratitude: An Evolutionary Journey to Awakening Your Spirit.* Carlsbad, CA: Hay House, 2007.

About the Author

Kathi Casey, EYRT, CPI, "The Healthy Boomer Body Expert," is a renowned health and wellness coach, Amazon bestselling author, trainer, popular speaker and radio show guest. She has appeared on Fox 23, *ABC-8 Evening News*, and *The Style Show,* and produces her own TV show, "To Your Health." She is a regular columnist for *The South Shore Senior News,* and *Boomer Living,* and has been published in *Life After 50* and *More* magazine. She's the founder of the Healthy Boomer Body Center in the Berkshires of Massachusetts. Her programs and products help end chronic back or neck pain, enhance the immune system, reduce stress, lower blood pressure, help you lose weight and *keep* it off— and laugh yourself well with *Laughing Meditation*! Her blog was ranked number 10 in NursingSchools.net's list of 50 top health blogs.

Kathi is a registered yoga teacher with Yoga Alliance (U.S. licensing agency), certified in Pilates from The Body College in Washington, D.C., and has continued her Pilates training with advanced courses. She is certified in acu-yoga through the Acupressure Institute in Berkeley, California, is trained in ayurvedic physical health and healing touch, and has studied somatics, qigong, meditation and more.

Kathi is healthier and more fit now than she was at age 20 and is passionate about sharing her tips and techniques with the world so that others can get the same results. For the last ten years, she's been teaching people up and down the East Coast how to take charge of their own health care— regardless of what Congress does! And she can help you too!

You can find all of Kathi's life changing health information at her website: www.HealthyBoomerBody.com

Books and DVD Programs by Kathi Casey, ERYT, CPI:

Get Rid of Sciatic Pain for Good!

Get Ready for Pilates®

Intermediate Pilates

Advanced Pilates

Pilates with Acupressure: An Immune System Boost

Acu-Yoga for Balancing Hormones: No More Hot Flashes

Get Off the Couch, Potato!: How to Lose Inches While Watching Oprah

All of Kathi's products and Coaching Services can be found at:
http://bit.ly/BackHealthNow

www.ingramcontent.com/pod-product-compliance
Lightning Source LLC
Chambersburg PA
CBHW060903280326
41934CB00007B/1162